ask

1000 most asked questions about
BEAUTY

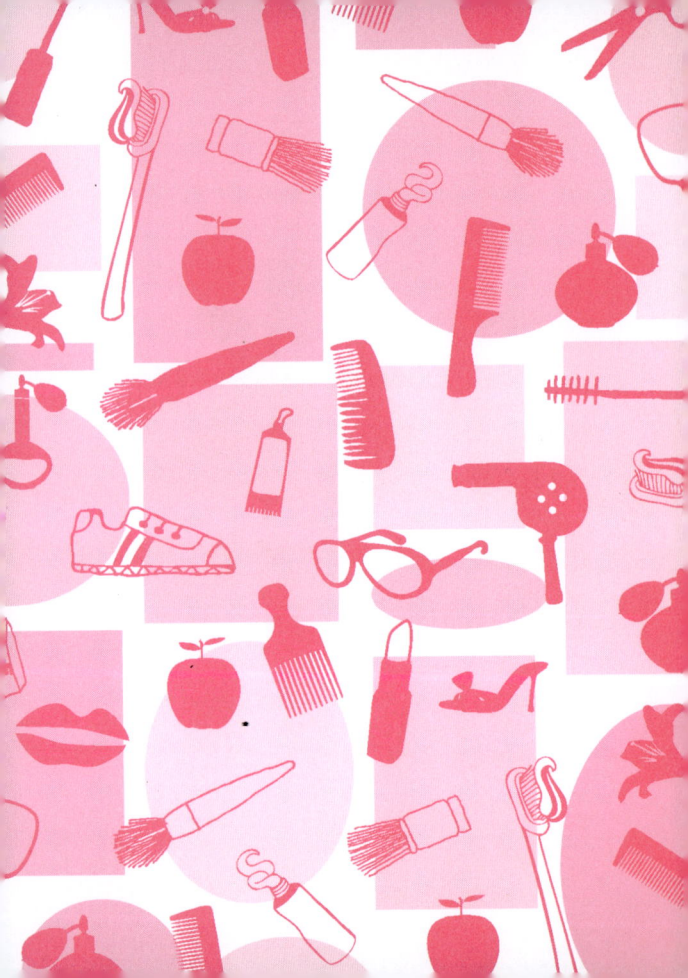

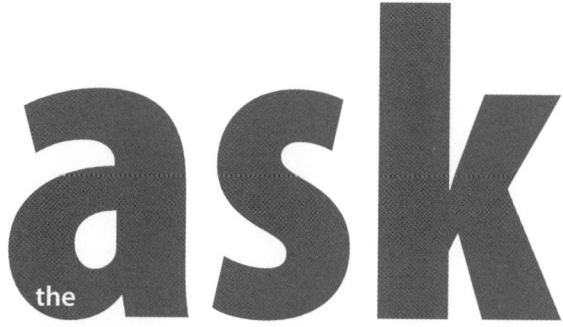

the ask
1000 most asked questions about
BEAUTY

Bella Blissett

spruce

An Hachette UK company
www.hachette.co.uk

First published in Great Britain in 2009 by Spruce, a division of Octopus Publishing Group Ltd.

Carmelite House, 50 Victoria Embankment, London, EC4Y 0DZ

This edition published in 2016

Copyright © Octopus Publishing Group Ltd 2009, 2016

Illustrations by Tim Wesson

Distributed in the US by Hachette Book Group, 1290 Avenue of the Americas, 4th and 5th Floors, New York, NY 10020

Distributed in Canada by Canadian Manda Group, 664 Annette St., Toronto, Ontario, Canada M6S 2C8

All rights reserved. No part of this work may be reproduced or utilized in any form or by any means, electronic or mechanical, including photocopying, recording, or by any information storage and retrieval system, without the prior written permission of the publisher.

ISBN 978-1-84601-520-5

Printed and bound in China

10 9 8 7 6 5 4 3 2 1

This book contains the opinions and ideas of the author. It is intended to provide helpful and informative material on the subjects addressed in this book and is sold with the understanding that the author and publisher are not engaged in rendering any kind of personal professional services in this book. The author and publisher disclaim all responsibility for any liability, loss, or risk, personal or otherwise, which is incurred as a consequence, directly or indirectly, of the use and application of any of the contents of this book.

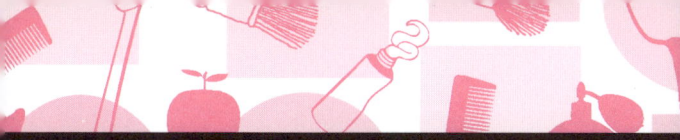

contents

Introduction	6
Five-minute SOS	8
Product savvy	34
Tools & techniques	94
Applying make-up	130
Treat yourself	162
Surgical intervention	206
Kitchen cupboard remedies	242
Alternative answers	270
Dress to impress	332
Travel tips	386
Myths & trivia	408
Index	442

Introduction

Have you ever wondered how to ward off wrinkles, crack cellulite, banish pimples or get a perfect complexion using placenta? Our pursuit of youth and beauty raises countless questions in our everyday lives. Women today are bombarded with information about how to achieve flawless skin, a great body, and glossy hair, yet most of it is conflicting advice. The beauty industry provides a never-ending stream of *miracle* products, but how do we know which ones really work? Does a hefty price tag guarantee results, or will something from our kitchen cupboards do just as well?

More than just a guide to the best lotions and potions, this book covers nutrition advice and fashion tricks to flatter your body, plus everything from ancient beauty rituals to the latest spa treatments and antiaging technology. It's the bluffer's guide to decoding product labels, applying make-up like a professional and knowing your Botox® from your Hydrafill®.

You may have an irritating niggle, or want products with a conscience, which are ethical, environmentally friendly, and chemical-free. If you can't seem to minimize your cosmetics on vacation, or if you've never known which make-up brushes to use when, read on. Here we cut through the minefield of beauty information, offering practical and effective solutions for your skin, hair, and body type, whether you want to grow old gracefully or use all the surgical help you can get.

Full of home remedies, quick fixes, clever tips, and strange myths (do pores really open and close?), this book presents the answers to the beauty questions that women of all ages want and need to know. For the times when you've got nothing to wear, you're having a bad hair day, or when you need a total image overhaul, let this be your guide.

Bella Blissett

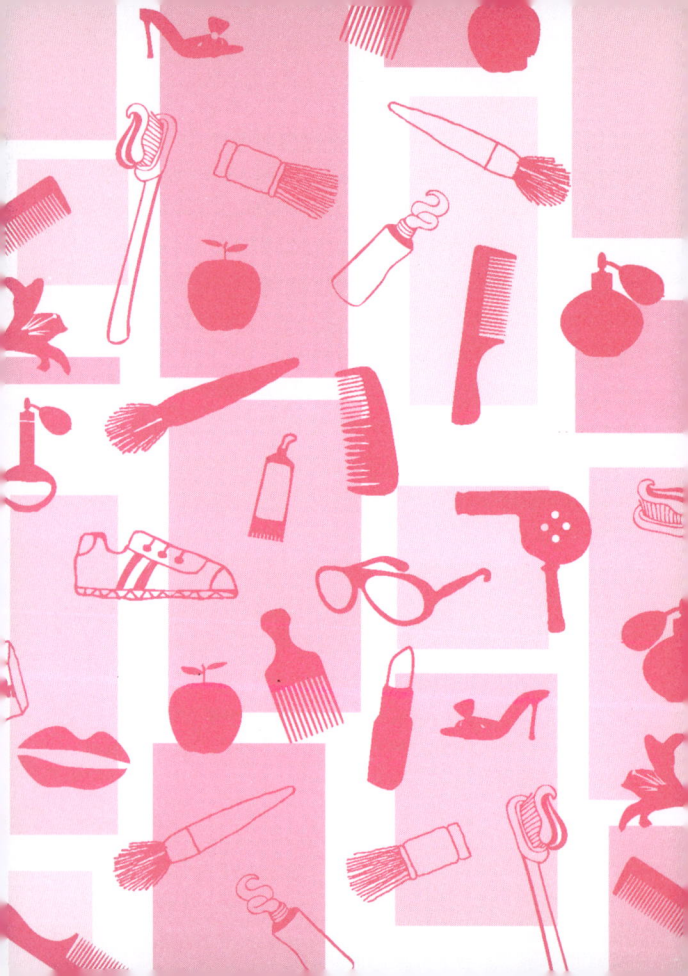

Five-minute SOS

"What can I do about the dark patches on my elbows and knees?"

Sprinkle sugar onto half a lemon and rub into the dark area to exfoliate and bleach the skin.

"What's an instant natural brightener for my skin?"

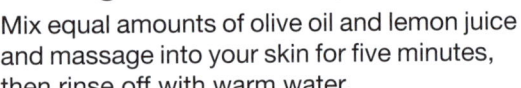

Mix equal amounts of olive oil and lemon juice and massage into your skin for five minutes, then rinse off with warm water.

"Is there any quick kitchen-cupboard remedy for dull skin?"

Mash up a crabapple, slather it on, and leave it for as long as you can. It contains natural alpha hydroxy acids to soften and exfoliate skin.

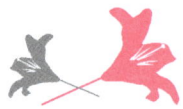

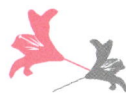

"What should I carry in my purse to give my skin some instant protection?"

Beauty editors swear by Elizabeth Arden's Eight Hour Cream, which offers intense moisturizing and helps protect against chapping. It's particularly good when you're going out in the cold or wind, or when you're flying.

"How can I get ink stains off my hands?"

Rub some toothpaste over the mark.

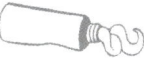

"What's a good way to remove fake tan streaks?"

Mix some lemon juice and salt together and use on a loofah to rub the streaky area.

"How can I make my skin glow when I don't have time to fake tan?"

Invest in some body shimmer and mix equal quantities with your usual body moisturizer. Slap some on before you get dressed: it will reflect the light and give you a glow without the tan.

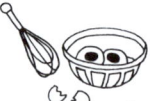

"Is there a quick, natural way to get a face-lift?"

Separate an egg, whisk the white until slightly stiffer then apply to the face for 20 minutes. Rinse off with warm water.

"What's an instant way of getting rid of dry skin on my face?"

When you're looking a bit flaky, exfoliation will remove the dead skin cells. If you've run out of exfoliator, add a small amount of sugar (brown if possible) to your usual cleansing wash and rub it gently over your face.

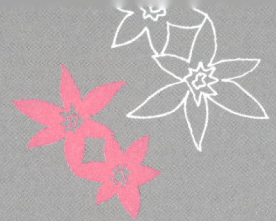

"How can I hide my wrinkles in a flash?"

If you've neither the time nor the inclination to use full-on fillers, the beauty industry has come up with *polyfillas* products that fill in wrinkles, putty-style. It may only be pasting over the cracks, but it beats caking on the powder, which only ends up highlighting your lines.

"How can I make a pimple look less visible?"

When a pimple appears from nowhere, dab a little nasal decongestant on it to constrict the blood vessels and reduce the eye-catching redness.

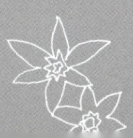

"Is there a quick-fix remedy for combating acne?"

Instead of wasting your money on expensive products, crush an aspirin with a few drops of water and dab on to the acne at bedtime. It's antibacterial and will reduce the redness.

"Can I treat a pimple and still wear make-up?"

Dab some apple cider vinegar onto the spot before applying your concealer.

"How can I stop the onset of a skin eruption?"

If you feel a monster bulging up from under the skin's surface, apply an ice cube to it several times a day to minimize the bulge.

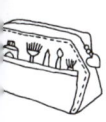

"I've forgotten my make-up bag. What's a quick pick-me-up for skin?"

In a make-up SOS, use that lip balm floating around in your purse and dab it along the cheek bones, in the inner corners of the eye, down the middle of the nose and on your mouth to add instant luminescence.

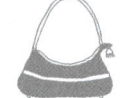

"If I only take one make-up product out with me, what should it be?"

If you can't take the whole lot, grab an all-in-one lip and cheek tint. This will give you a lip stain and blush and it's surprising how a little color can add radiance to your face while detracting from any flaws.

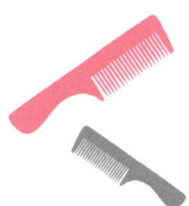

"How can I give my tired make-up an instant lift?"

A smudge of blush on the apples of your cheeks and a quick lick of mascara will do wonders.

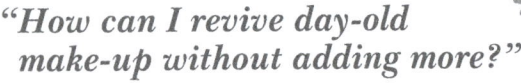

"How can I revive day-old make-up without adding more?"

Instead of caking on more, sweep a small amount of moisturizer beneath your eyes and on any uneven patches to smooth out your skin tone and redistribute the make-up you applied earlier.

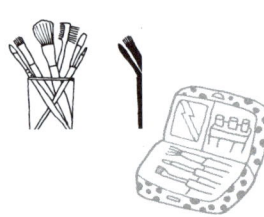

"How can I fix the oily patches that ruin my make-up in summer?"

Instead of applying more make-up (which will only look thick and flaky), carry a packet of cosmetic blotting paper around in your purse and mop up the oil when you need to. Follow it with a very light dusting of translucent powder.

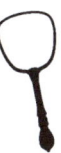

"How do I fix an excess blush emergency?"

If you go overboard with the blush, don't be tempted to use make-up remover, because you'll only ruin your carefully prepared base. Instead, use a cotton ball to brush away the excess. Then apply a layer of translucent powder to tone down your flaming cheeks.

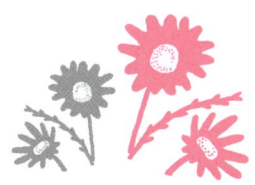

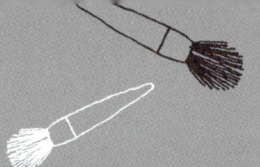

"How can I patch up my false lashes when they start to fall off?"

If one side starts to drop, apply a thin coat of mascara to the lashes below and use it to stick the false ones back on.

"What's a quick-fix way of refreshing tired eyes?"

Mix up a bottle containing equal quantities of rosewater and mineral water and keep it in your fridge. When tiredness strikes, soak a couple of cotton balls in the mixture and place them on your eyes for a few minutes.

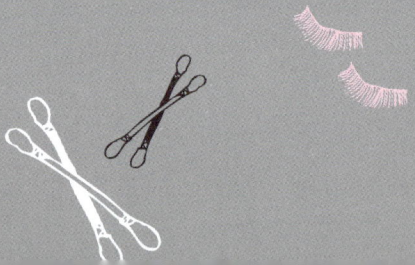

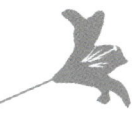

"How can I stop my eye shadow from flaking onto my cheeks when I apply it?"

Reverse your make-up routine and apply your eye shadow before your foundation and concealer. Also, ensure that you always knock the excess powder off your shadow brush before application.

"I'm in a hurry and my mascara is all lumpy in the tube. Help!"

If you find your mascara clumping at the bottom of the tube, let it rest in some warm water for a few minutes to heat the mixture and liquefy it once more.

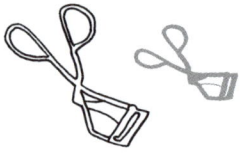

"How can I curl my lashes quickly?"

If you've no time to fiddle around with eyelash curlers, run a teaspoon under warm water, then press it to the base of your lashes for a few seconds.

"How can I give my lashes an instant boost?"

Apply one coat of mascara, followed by one of primer, then a final sweep of mascara. It's the make-up artist's secret to lashes that go on forever.

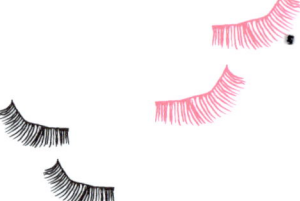

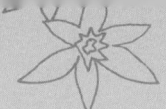

"What's the best brush for doing smoky eyes fast?"

Use a wide, contoured brush with soft bristles that come almost to a point in the middle. It's the perfect shape for blending shadow in the outer corner of the eye and into the crease.

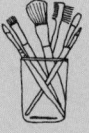

"What's an instant fix for creased eye shadow?"

Resist the temptation to put more shadow on top. Instead, use some Vaseline® and the tip of your finger to even it out again.

"Is there anything I can do to hide my saggy eyelids?"

Make like Japanese women and use a Mezaik Eyelid Crease Maker: a stretchy strip that fits over the eyelid giving one defined crease and an otherwise smooth appearance. From www.naturaljapanesebeauty.com.

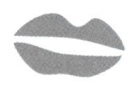

"How can I tame my brows when I haven't got the time to get to the beauty salon?"

Sweep a colored brow gel over them to fill in gaps and keep stray hairs in place.

"How do I fix my messy brows when I haven't got any special products?"

Messy brows make for a messy face, so when you've only minutes to spare, smear some Vaseline® on your toothbrush and use it to smooth stray hairs into place.

"How can I fix a broken lipstick?"

Set the broken bit aside and place the remainder of the lipstick in the tube under a naked flame to soften (not melt) it. Weld your stray piece back on and leave to cool. Lipstick saved.

"I'm all out of lip balm. How can I cure my dry lips fast?"

Rub a small amount of butter into your lips to smooth them and add a subtle sheen.

"How can I make my lips look instantly fuller?"
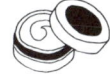

Add a few drops of peppermint oil to your usual lip balm to get plumper lips in seconds.

"How can I freshen my breath naturally?"

Chew cardamom seeds or parsley leaves.

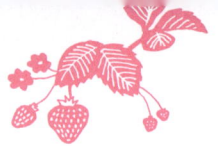

"How can I make an instant natural whitener for my teeth?"

Crush some fresh strawberries and rub them over your teeth, allowing the seeds to help polish off stains.

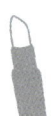

"How can I make my teeth look brighter?"

Pick a lipstick with blue undertones to highlight your teeth.

"How can I get a celebrity smile?"

The Snap-on-Smile® is here to save the day. After a dentist has taken a mold of your teeth, you can ask for your new smile to resemble that of a particular celeb. You'll be given a plastic set of teeth to slot on over your own at a moment's notice when you need a perfect Hollywood smile.

"What clears a blocked nose fast?"

Sniff some marjoram, peppermint, or rosemary oil.

"What's the best way to hide my raw nose when I have a cold?"

Find a moisturizing concealer that contains ingredients such as vitamin E, jojoba oil, and beeswax to replenish the dry skin. A slightly blue undertone will also balance out the redness.

"How can I remove deodorant marks from my clothes?"

Don't splash yourself with water because you'll only create enormous sweatlike patches. Use a facial cleansing wipe to remove them instantly.

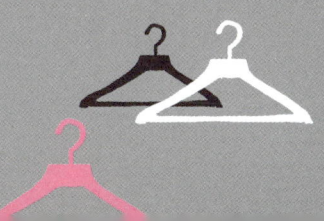

"How can I remove the stains on my white jeans in a hurry?"

Don't even think about using wet toilet paper. Carry some white chalk in your handbag for emergency touch-ups until you have time to wash them.

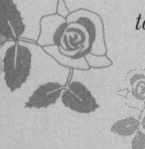

"I've run out of shaving cream. Is there anything I can use instead?"

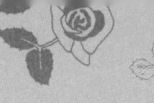

When you've got legs like a yeti and no time to run down to the drugstore, try slathering on some hair conditioner, or even some olive oil, before shaving to protect from cuts and leave your legs super smooth.

"How can I zap stress?"

Massage some lavender oil into your temples and take deep breaths until you feel calmer.

"How can I give myself an instant mood boost?"

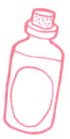

Take some deep breaths while holding a bottle of energizing bergamot or frankincense oil just beneath your nose.

"How do I thin clogged-up nail polish?"

Add a few drops of nail polish remover to the polish and shake the bottle well before applying.

"What's the best way to stop nail varnish from drying up in the pot?"

Keep it in the refrigerator.

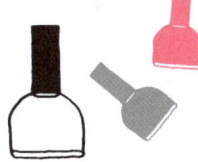

"How do I tackle a snagged nail?"

If you're on a night out with no nail file, grab a box of matches from the bar and use the ignition strip instead.

"How can I keep my nails dirt-free when I'm gardening?"

If you're finger-deep in a flower bed (or anywhere else with a lot of dirt), scrape your nails over a bar of soap before starting, to stop the dirt from getting underneath them.

"When's the best time to paint my fingernails?"

Do it last thing before walking out the door, after putting your coat on and scrabbling around for your keys in your bag. The cold air will dry it as you travel to your destination. Never do it just before a bath because the hot water makes it more prone to chipping.

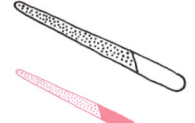

"How can I stop my cuticles from splitting in winter?"

Splitting tends to occur when the skin dries out in the winter winds and moisture-sapping central heating. Carry some Vaseline® or cocoa butter lip balm around with you and apply it to both your lips and cuticles throughout the day to kill two beauty birds with one stone.

"How can I stop my fake tan from staining my nails yellow?"

Rub some Vaseline® on and around your nails to stop the color from taking in these areas.

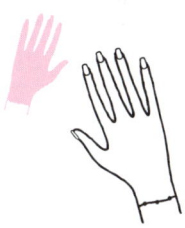

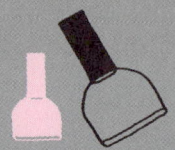

"Is there a way to rescue smudged nails?"

Instead of starting all over again, dip a finger from the other hand into some nail polish remover and gently rub it over the smudged nail. Leave it to dry, paint one layer of your colored polish over it, then finish with a topcoat.

"I'm wearing open-toe shoes; how can I fix my ugly toenails fast?"

Always keep a set of false toenails in your bathroom to be stuck on in emergencies.

"Is there a quick fix for lank hair?"

Boost your locks by applying a little white wine vinegar while you're in the shower. Leave for a couple of minutes and rinse.

"How do I tame flyaway hair in a hurry?"
Get rid of the static by passing a silk scarf over your hair.

"How can I cover greasy blonde roots?"
Forget talc (you'll look gray) and use some loose powder from your make-up bag instead. The color is likely to be closer to the color of both your scalp and hair and it will help soak up excess oil.

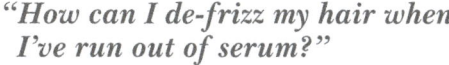

"How can I de-frizz my hair when I've run out of serum?"

Try rubbing some of your usual hand cream or lip balm into your palms, then smooth over your hair to flatten stray ends and banish frizz.

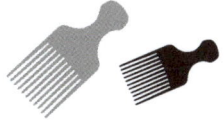

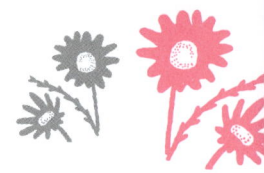

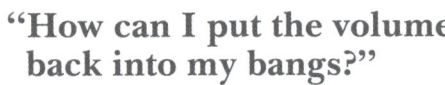

"How can I put the volume back into my bangs?"

When you wake up with a flat mop, apply a small amount of volumizing mousse and roll your bangs in Velcro rollers. Blast with hot followed by cold air.

"How can I get away with day-old hair?"

Use some of the hair-refresher products on the market, either wet or dry shampoos, to soak up any excess oil at the root. Blast the roots with a dryer while turning your head upside down to give them a good-as-new volume boost.

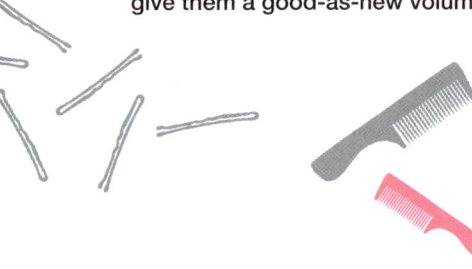

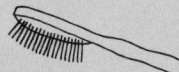

"What are my purse essentials when I'm dashing out the door?"

Do the ten-point checklist: keys, cellphone, wallet, Vaseline® (for lips and brow tidying), hand cream (to double up as face moisturizer and hair smoother), make-up (concealer, blush, lip and cheek tint, and mascara are the minimum), water, chewing gum, hair brush, plus safety pins and Hollywood tape (for fashion emergencies).

"How can I get a blow-dry in a hurry?"

Some clothes shops are now introducing blow-dry bars. You turn up (without having made an appointment), select from one of the custom blow-dries (they'll show you a picture), and walk out looking fabulous.

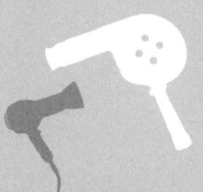

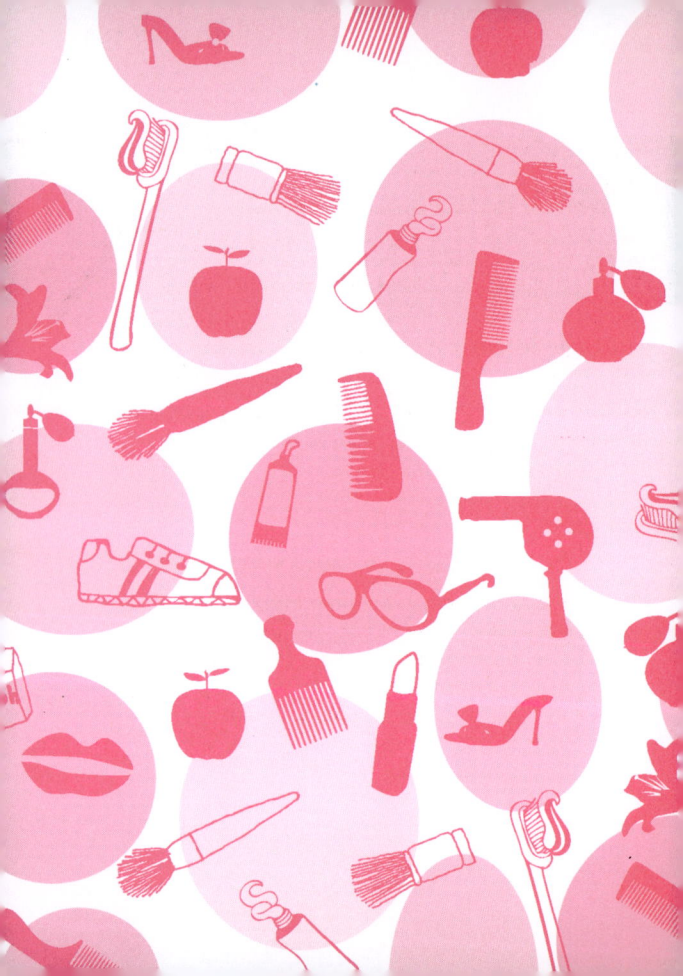

Product savvy

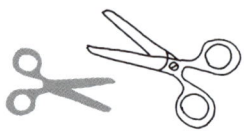

"Should I stick to one product line?"

The manufacturers will tell you that the products from a brand have been made to complement each other, increasing their efficacy. However, you know your skin better than the advertisers, so if it suits you to shop around, do so.

"Which are the best websites for ordering beauty products online?"

For a wide variety of supplement and skincare brands, www.victoriahealth.com is your best bet. If you want electrical beauty appliances or make-up, including some quirkier ranges than those sold in the department stores, try www.hqhair.com.

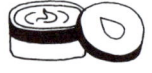

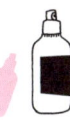

"Are fragrance-free products safer?"

Artificial fragrances, which are added to cosmetics, can be harmful. There are no laws governing the labeling of products with *fragrance-free* or *unscented*, so even these products may contain nasties to mask the fatty smell of soap. Check the small print for individual ingredients.

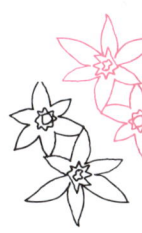

"How can I tell if a brand is made ethically or not?"

Check out its ethiscore, a rating given by the Ethical Consumer Research Association for sustainability, humane working conditions, animal testing policy, and commitment to environmentally friendly processes. Visit www.ethiscore.org to find a brand's rating.

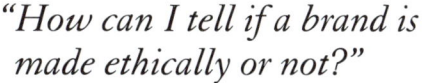

"How can I look after my skin without harming the environment?"

Palm oil is used in many cosmetics and contributes to the deforestation of Indonesia, the destruction of orangutan habitats and the burning of peatlands, resulting in greenhouse gas emissions. If you want to do something to help save the planet, look for brands that only use palm oil from sustainable sources.

"How often do I need to throw out my cosmetics?"

Different products have a different shelf life, but in general, anything used on the eye area should be thrown out every four to six months, moisturizers and foundations after about a year and powders after two or three years. Natural products tend to spoil more rapidly, because they don't usually contain preservatives.

"How can I make my cosmetics last longer?"

Store them somewhere cool and dark and always ensure you replace the lids. Never add water to products that have dried out because you could introduce bacteria, causing skin breakouts or eye infections.

"Does organic really mean organic?"

There are no laws restricting the use of the word *organic*, and many products labeled in this way are still full of chemicals, preservatives, and pesticides. If you do buy into the claim that truly organic ingredients contain more potent skin-rejuvenating ingredients, make sure the product is accredited by an organic organization, to ensure it has had minimal processing and contains no pesticides or genetically modified ingredients.

"What should an authentic organic product contain?"

It should contain at least 95% natural ingredients, or ingredients derived from natural products. In 2008 the Natural Products Association launch the new standard that defines natural and only products that display their official seal are guaranteed to be certified natural.

"What's a humectant?"

Anything that promotes the retention of water. Glycerin is a natural humectant.

"What's a surfactant?"

Meaning *surface-active agent*, this is an important element in cosmetics that stops oil- and water-based ingredients from separating. Surfactants come in the form of detergents and foaming agents in facial cleansers.

"What's so bad about parabens?"

They are toxic, synthetic preservatives that have been known to contribute to asthma, eczema, and rashes. These endocrine-disrupting chemicals (EDCs) get absorbed into the blood stream and disrupt the hormonal system; traces of them have been found in cancerous tumors. They may be labeled as methyl, ethyl, propyl, butyl, and hydroxy methyl benozoates.

"What are the really nasty ingredients I should avoid?"

Ingredients that have been directly linked to cancer or hormonal disruption, including green3, blue1, padimate-O, sodium hydroxymethyl-glycinate, toluene, xylene, BHT, propylene glycol, crystalline silica, coal tar dyes, talc, DEA and TEA (diethanolamine and triethanolamine), pthalates, parabens, and formaldehyde.

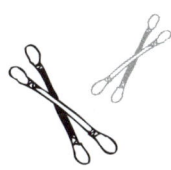

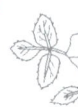

"Which ingredients are safe?"

Despite the hype surrounding potentially dangerous ingredients, there are also many natural, nonharmful ones. Titanium and zinc oxides are natural minerals found in eye shadows, foundation, and many products containing sunscreen. Beeswax and jojoba are found in lipsticks, glosses, and concealer, while karite butter (also known as shea butter) is a natural fat extracted from the shea tree.

"Is lanolin completely safe?"

Because lanolin is a natural oil taken from sheep's fleeces at shearing, people often assume it's risk-free. It may, however, contain pesticides applied to the wool, which can cause adverse reactions in the skin.

"Is the alcohol-free *label foolproof?"*

This labeling refers to ethyl alcohol, which has a strong drying effect on the skin. The product may still contain fatty alcohols, such as stearyl alcohol, which is an emollient used to soften the skin, but is much less likely to cause irritation.

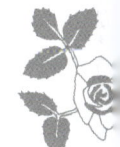

"Are *preservative-free* products better for my skin?"

Preservatives are there for a reason: to make the product last longer and protect against contamination from microbes. Without the preservatives, your skin can be vulnerable to infection, but too many preservatives and you may get an allergic reaction. The trick is to find a balance between the two.

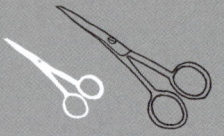

"I've always used the same products. Is there any reason to change?"

Aside from curiosity, it depends on how well you rate your products. The needs of your skin will change throughout your lifetime, so trying some new products can sometimes get better results.

"Is there a budget-buy product that celebrities swear by?"

If you're strapped for cash but still want glowing skin, look no further than Johnson's Baby Oil. Jessica Alba is rumored to mix a pea-sized amount with her daily moisturizer to give it a healthy shimmer.

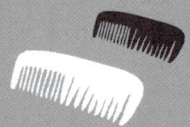

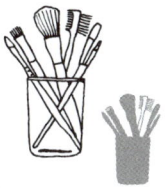

"What type of make-up brushes are best?"

Brushes with natural bristles are best for powder. To dodge the price tag of natural make-up brushes, try looking in your local artists' supply store. They will have a similar thing at a fraction of the price.

"Is it a good idea to test products in stores?"

Tester samples can be tried by hundreds of people and are a haven for bacteria. Ask for a sealed sachet to take away or, at the very least, avoid testing products for lips and eyes.

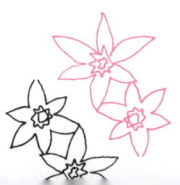

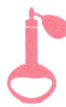

"Which cult beauty products should no woman be without?"

Chanel No. 5, to smell classic, not cloying; Elizabeth Arden Eight Hour Cream for ultimate moisture; YSL Touche Eclat for under-eye circles; Vaseline® for a multitude of beauty dilemmas; B Never Too Busy to be Beautiful lipstick for crimson lips; and Crème de la Mer hand and body crème for youthful skin all over.

"Is it safe to use make-up that has melted?"

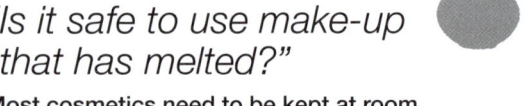

Most cosmetics need to be kept at room temperature or even in the refrigerator. Overheating can cause changes in the chemical ingredients, so it's best to get replacements as soon as you can.

"How can I tell if a product has been tested on animals?"

Watch out for the jumping rabbit symbol on your cosmetics bottles; it means that the product has been approved by the International Humane Cosmetics Standards and has undergone no animal testing.

"Essential oils are natural: does that mean they are completely safe?"

Not at all. Essential oils can be extremely powerful, especially if they are not diluted. It's better to seek the advice of a professional if you're new to them.

"Are essential oils safe for everyone?"

They should be avoided in the first three months of pregnancy, and after that time you should seek advice from a doctor. They should not be used on young children, and breastfeeding mothers should avoid them to prevent passing them onto their babies.

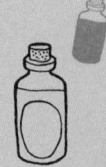

"Is there a product I can use from sustainable resources?"

Hemp oil is perfect. Not only is it rich in the essential oils that your skin requires for nourishment, but the hemp crop is also sustainable and simple to grow, requiring no fertilizers or pesticides.

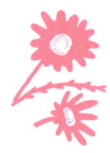

"What one product can transform my day make-up to night make-up?"

A wet-dry foundation dusts on dry for a lighter daytime finish, and can be sponged on wet for heavier coverage that will last when you're partying the night away.

"What should I do if my preferred product has been discontinued?"

There's not much you can do about this one. Try writing to the manufacturer to find out if they still have some, have reissued it under a different name, or if the product is merely being discontinued temporarily.

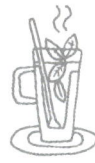 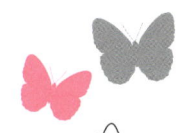

"What is an antioxidant and why is it good for my skin?"

Antioxidants are nutrients that ward off damage from free radicals: the reactive molecules that cause both internal and external aging.

"When should I start using antiaging products?"

Up to about the age of 30, you should stick to protecting your skin in basic ways: ensure it's well moisturized and apply an SPF and an EPF (environmental protection factor) against harmful environmental factors. Leave it until later to go heavy with the collagen boosters and line erasers.

 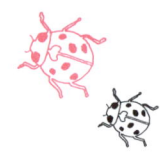

"What are the key ingredients I should look for in an antiaging product?"

Dermatologists recommend co-enzyme Q10, carotenoids, vitamins C and E, flavonoids, idebenone, ferulic acid, and lycopene. Hyaluronic acid is another wonder ingredient that skincare experts swear by.

"What are AHAs?"

Alpha hydroxy acids, derived from fruit or milk sugars. They work to exfoliate the skin and promote the growth of new cells, giving a more youthful complexion. Glycolic acid comes from sugar cane, lactic acid from milk, malic acid from apples and pears, citric acid from oranges and lemons, and tartaric acid from grapes.

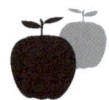 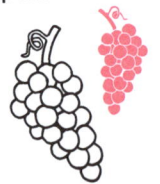

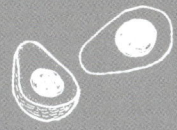

"Are AHAs suitable for all skin types?"

Beware the influence of advertising. AHAs are marketed as miracle skin ingredients but they're often too harsh for sensitive skins and unnecessary for young skins. They may be exfoliating agents, but too much scraping away the upper layers of skin can leave it more exposed to environmental damage and aging.

"Can products really eliminate fine lines and wrinkles?"

Unless it's a filler, fat implant, face-lift, or skin peel, then forget it. Nothing you apply topically will erase wrinkles completely.

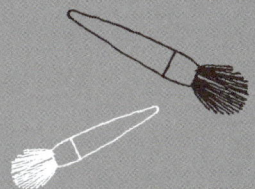

"Is there a product with similar effects to Botox®?"

No topical products will ever have the same effect as an injection, but the beauty industry's new hi-tech miracle-workers can produce a similar effect in the short term. These work by filling the wrinkles, increasing collagen production, and using light-deflecting polymers to conceal flaws.

"Can you get the Botox® effect in a bottle?"

One of the brands to come close is Hydroderm®, a selection of products from antiwrinkle and eye serums to lip volumizers. The makers claim to have discovered an effective way of transporting vital ingredients to skin cells to combat lines and wrinkles.

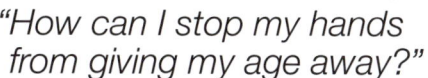

"How can I stop my hands from giving my age away?"

If your face is as smooth as a baby's bottom but your hands are looking a little on the leathery side, invest in a pair of professional salon-heated manicure mitts (try Jessica or Babyliss). Slather on a thick, oil-based moisturizer, don the mitts, and relax in front of the television. The heat helps the moisturizer to penetrate more deeply and restore your hands to softness.

"What can I do about my age spots?"

Products containing hydroquinone inhibit the production of melanin, which is responsible for these dark patches. Over-the-counter creams contain concentrations of 0.5 to 2 percent, but stronger doses are available from doctors.

"Every week there seems to be a new miracle product or beauty pill on the market. What should I do?"

There's no guarantee that any product will ward off the signs of aging, but if you want to cover your bases invest in some cosmeceuticals, a cross between cosmetics and pharmaceuticals that work to improve both your body's inner health and external appearance. Mineral make-up brands such as Mineral FX, Barefaced Beauty and Lily Lolo all contain zinc oxides, which have healing properties for the skin, act as anti-inflammatories, and provide a natural sunscreen.

"What's co-enzyme Q10?"

In many people over the age of 30, levels of co-enzyme Q10 are below optimum, lessening the body's ability to produce collagen. This antioxidant is used in anti-aging products to help boost skin repair and rejuvenation and smooth out your lines.

"How can I keep my chest and cleavage firm?"

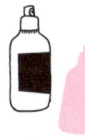

There are products that claim to produce similar results to having your breasts lifted surgically. These contain peptides, pro-collagen wonders, and other miracle ingredients, but don't believe everything you read on a label. Always keep your chest and breasts well moisturized by applying cream with long, upward sweeping movements and never go out in the sun without an SPF.

"Are there any antiaging wonder ingredients I should know about?"

Idebenone is an organic compound and antioxidant that has been shown to be more successful at mopping up the free radicals that contribute to aging than many other ingredients on the market.

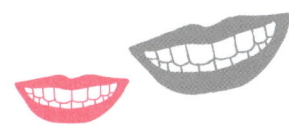

> *"Is it true that antiaging creams don't penetrate the skin deep enough to have an effect?"*

According to some experts, antiaging products are only absorbed into the upper layer of the skin (the epidermis). Some of the new, high-tech products now claim to penetrate to the dermal-epidermal junction (DEJ), the area joining the epidermis with the underlying dermis. As we age, the surface area of this junction layer is reduced so it is deprived of adequate nutrients to rebuild and repair itself, resulting in deep wrinkles.

> *"What are pentapeptides?"*

These long-chain amino acids act as chemical messengers inside the body. Originally discovered for their ability to assist in wound healing, they have been found to help stimulate the production of collagen to support the skin's structure and keep it looking youthful.

"Which ingredients help mature skin?"

Pro-xylane, an antiaging molecule used in products targeted at women of menopausal age, comes from a compound found in Eastern European beech trees. It stimulates the function of the skin's extra-cellular matrix, which provides a means of communication between the cells and helps it maintain its structure and shape.

"Could stem cells be the answer to eternal youth?"

Whichever side of the stem-cell debate you stand on, they could help fight wrinkles. Scientists are working on a way of using stem cells from your own body to help rebuild and repair the skin, but it will be illegal in many parts of the world.

"Do cellulite-busting creams really work?"

The ingredients of these so-called miracle products vary, but all contain some sort of moisturizing agent. This helps to a degree, because dehydrated skin generally looks thinner, making those fatty pockets more noticeable. Maintaining moisture levels will certainly make your orange-peel less obvious.

"Is it true that you should never use soap on your face?"

The detergents in soap can affect the delicate pH balance of your facial skin and strip it of its protective liquid film, leaving it dry. Soap can also encourage the growth of bacteria, causing breakouts and irritation. Stick to a gentle natural cleanser that suits your skin type.

"How do I combat dry, irritated skin?"

If you're exfoliating too often (more than twice a week) or using products containing retin-A, cut back and instead use a deeply hydrating mask every day until the irritation subsides.

"What's a quick way to remove make-up without damaging my skin?"

You may want to remove your make-up, but you need to avoid stripping the skin of its natural protective layer. Daily cleansing has a tendency to leave skin feeling tight and dry. Nude Skincare's natural cleansing oil (www.nudeskincare.com) rubs on like a rich balm, then turns milky when you add a few drops of water to your face. Because it's free from detergent and chemicals, you can sweep it over your eyes too. The added omega-3s and vitamin E in the cleanser will nourish and protect your skin while you cleanse.

"What's the difference between serum and moisturizer?"

Moisturizer is an emulsion that hydrates the skin, while serum is lighter and runnier and contains "active" ingredients that claim to do something extra such as reducing wrinkles or brightening the complexion.

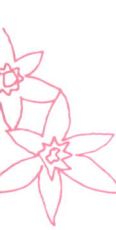

"What are liposomes?"

Liposomes are the couriers of skin care. They help transfer active ingredients in skin products to the cells, making them more effective.

"What on earth are ceramides?"

Ceramides are part of the skin's lipid layer, which helps it retain moisture and keeps it looking plump and youthful. A drop in ceramide levels causes dehydration and an increase in the appearance of wrinkles. Manufacturers now make synthetic versions to help reverse this process and the resulting signs of aging.

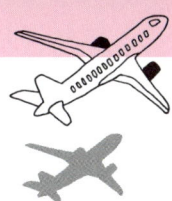

"What can I do to protect my skin from pollutants in the city?"

We know about the dangers of the sun, but many of us are less aware of the harmful effects of other environmental factors and pollutants. Cosmetics companies are now making products with an SPF and an EPF (environmental protection factor). These protect not only against sun damage but also against wind, pollution, and ozone, all of which play a part in skin aging.

"What should a skin-lightening product contain?"

Look out for kojic acid.

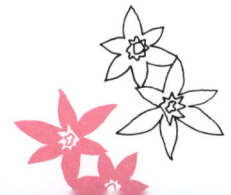

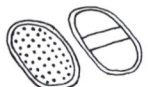

"How do I know which exfoliator is right for me?"

Match the particles in your scrub to the size of your pores. A chunky exfoliator is good for those with large pores while something more subtle will do for smaller pores.

"I have very sensitive skin. What's the best way to treat it gently?"

Don't use products with astringents such as menthol and alcohol, never splash very hot water on your face, and avoid facials that include steaming or extraction (squeezing the pores). Also avoid rough scrubs or abrasive cleansing cloths and always pat, rather than rub, your face dry.

"Are there any topical creams to target spider veins?"

Try applying some horse chestnut cream (available from health food stores). It is said to strengthen capillaries.

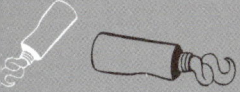

"What's the best thing to use on stretch marks?"

Marketed as being better than Botox®, Strivectin™ comes in a tube. Its magic seems to lie in the peptide formula that helps to soften deep lines such as stretch marks.

"Should I change my beauty regime during pregnancy?"

You might want to avoid hair depilatories, all-over-scalp hair dyes, and nail polish containing formaldehyde, some of the cosmetics known to be jam-packed with chemicals and potential allergens.

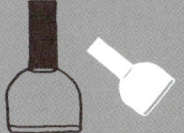

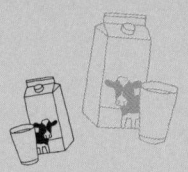

"Are there any product lines dedicated to pregnant women?"

Brands such as Mama Mio (www.mamamio.co.uk) specialize in products free from paraben and formaldehyde, but tackle everything from the lack of skin elasticity to the aches, pains, and itchiness that come with pregnancy.

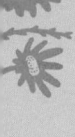

"What's the difference between alpha and beta hydroxy acids?"

Both acids, derived from fruit or milk, act as an exfoliant on the skin. But while alphas are only soluble in water, betas can penetrate sebum in pores to clear away dead skin that has built up inside. Betas are therefore better for oily skin.

"How can I stop my skin from getting so weather-beaten in winter?"

All that buffeting by cold winter wind and rain can leave even the most porcelain of complexions looking ruddy. The petroleum jelly in Vaseline® is one of the best (and cheapest) ways of creating a barrier against moisture loss, which causes dryness and irritation.

"How can I tell if a product is really working?"

Because you see your reflection every day, you may not notice subtle changes in your skin. If you really want to put a product through its paces, try using it for one month on one side of your face only.

"What should a good soap contain?"

Look for soaps with extra fat-based ingredients, such as lanolin, cocoa butter, or coconut oil, to help keep the skin moisturized.

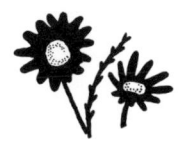

"Do I really need separate day and night creams?"

While day creams should provide a barrier to moisture loss, protect against sun and environmental damage, and work in tandem with your make-up, the role of a night cream is different. Richer in texture, they usually contain higher concentrations of active ingredients designed to repair the skin while we sleep. A night cream is too heavy for the day and a day cream won't give you the full replenishing benefits at night.

"How do I know if I'm using the right product for my skin type?"

It's more a case of knowing what's not right. Anything that leaves your face feeling tingly, stinging, or tight is too harsh for your skin type and you should change to something gentler.

"Can I use the same products on my face as I do on my body?"

Facial skin is not only thinner and more delicate than that on the body, but it is also more acidic because the orifices (mouth, nostrils, eyes, and ears) require extra defense from harmful germs. Because the two have different needs, it makes sense to use different products to treat them.

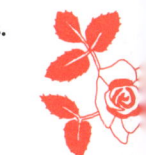

"How can I protect my skin from sun damage?"

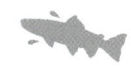

Try astaxanthin, a natural color carotenoid pigment and antioxidant found in oily foods, such as salmon.

"Which cosmetic ingredient is responsible for stimulating collagen production?"

Many pro-collagen products contain copper peptides, which not only boost the skin's elasticity but also assist the action of antioxidants and promote wound healing.

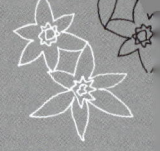
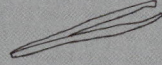

"What on earth is 'advanced antioxidant technology'?"

This can also be labeled as AO+ and is a flashy term skincare companies put on their labels to refer to a delivery system, which they claim helps antioxidants act more effectively on the skin.

"What should I look for in a facemask for oily skin?"

Kaolin is a fine natural clay from Mount Kaolin in China. It has been used for many years to draw out toxins and impurities from the skin and dry up excess sebum.

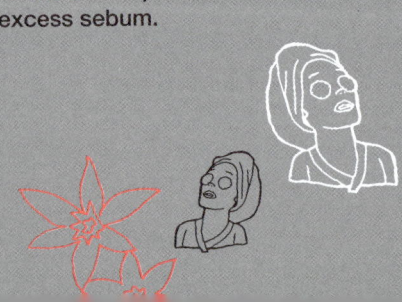

"Should I use an oil-based cleanser on my shiny skin?"

Perversely enough, you should use an oil-based cleanser to dissolve the excess sebum on your skin. Avoid harsh, alcohol-based cleansers, which will irritate your skin.

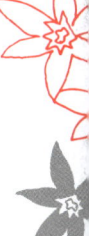

"How can I treat uneven skin pigmentation?"

Look for products that contain natural brightening agents such as mulberry, licorice, or bearberry, plus vitamin C and lactic acid.

"What wonder products are available for uneven skin pigmentation?"

The new cosmeceuticals contain niacin (a B vitamin), a so-called miracle ingredient for making patchy skin more even in tone.

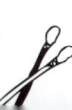

"Are there any new *superfood* ingredients I should look for?"

If you've done pomegranates and are sick of blueberries, seek out elderberry-based products. Scientists believe that a compound called anthocyanin, which gives the berry its color, can improve the skin's structure and appearance when applied topically.

"What are chili peppers doing in skin care products?"

Chili peppers are now being used in products for their ability to increase blood flow to the skin's surface and allow for a more efficient absorption of the product's antiaging ingredients.

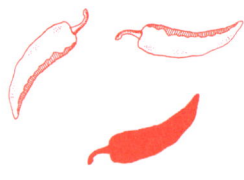

"What are the A-listers using on their skin?"

Doing the Hollywood rounds is pyratine-6, a derivative of kinetin (a plant hormone that promotes cell division). Pyrantine-6 has traditionally been used to treat acne and rosacea.

"What are the new trends in skin care?"

Look for "instant face-lifts," products developed by space agency scientists and cosmetic chemists, which claim to make a noticeable difference to your skin in a matter of minutes.

"What are the new antioxidant ingredients?"

The coffee berry (a fruit of the coffee plant) is said by some to be one of the richest sources of antioxidants because it grows near the Equator at high altitudes where the sun's oxidizing rays are strongest.

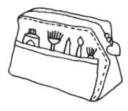

"Can make-up ever be beneficial to my skin?"

Manufacturers are developing new antiaging make-up products, such as lipsticks with collagen to replump lips and eye shadows that lift sagging eyes.

"What type of cleanser is best for my skin type?"

For oily or acne-prone skin, use a gentle or foam cleanser to dissolve excess oil on the skin's surface. For normal skin, use a lotion containing mild detergents and moisturizers. For dry or sensitive skin, try a rich, creamy cleanser for ultimate moisture, also good for older skins.

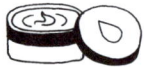

"Should I use an acid or alkaline cleanser?"

Many soap-based washes are highly alkaline and strip the skin of its naturally acidic protective layer. Choose a cleanser or wash near to the skin's pH (4.5 to 5.5) to clean your face without destroying this barrier.

"Does *pure* or *natural* on a product label mean that it is entirely safe for my skin?"

If you think those two words mean a product is chemical free, think again. In fact, they could only contain 2 percent natural ingredients; the other 98 percent could be entirely chemicals. Even natural ingredients will have been processed before they are bottled, and just because something has come from nature doesn't mean that it can't irritate your skin.

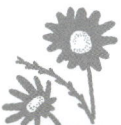

"Are there any natural ingredients I should look for in skin care?"

Green tea, seaweed, and natural fruit extracts are all thought to have antiaging properties. Frankincense oil has also been used for centuries to soothe and repair the skin.

"What's tocopherol?"

Sounds suspicious, but it's actually only vitamin E, an antioxidant used in many face creams.

"What's an emollient?"

Emollients act as a barrier to moisture loss, helping to keep the skin hydrated.

"How can I tell which products will be suitable for my sensitive skin?"

In general, the fewer the ingredients, the less likely a product is to cause irritation.

"How can I clear up the acne on my back?"

Just like your face, your back needs special attention. Use a long-handled body brush and Dead Sea Salt to exfoliate twice a week and rub gently in a circular movement to remove the dead skin cells that can block pores. Follow with a cleanser containing antibacterial properties, such as tea tree oil, and moisturize with body lotion.

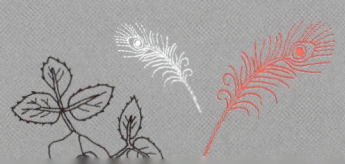

"Will acne formulas really stop me from getting pimples?"

These creams only treat visible acne. Many pimples form under the skin for weeks before coming out, so it's by no means a failsafe way to a clear complexion.

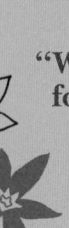

"Which types of products are good for skin that's prone to breakouts?"

Anything that markets itself as being "non-comedogenic" or "non-occlusive," meaning that they do not clog pores.

"What type of facemask should I buy to target my pimples and blackheads?"

Self-warming facemasks heat up when applied to the skin to open the pores and draw out impurities that cause pimples and blackheads. Look for one that contains charcoal, which acts as a magnet to impurities, leaving you with clearer pores and skin.

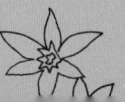

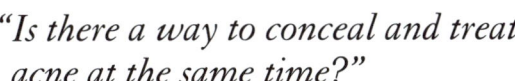

"Is there a way to conceal and treat acne at the same time?"

Choose a concealer that contains salicylic acid or benzoyl peroxide to promote healing.

"What kind of facial wash should I use on blackheads?"

Look for one with salicylic acid or alpha hydroxy acids, which exfoliate the skin and help to remove pore-clogging debris.

"How can I hide the acne on my back and chest?"

It's not just faces that can benefit from foundation. Use a make-up spray foundation designed especially for the body to cover up your blemishes. Don't be tempted to use your facial concealer because the skin on your face will be a different shade to that on your body.

"Can I treat toenail infections naturally?"

Check out brands, such as Foot Essentials, which make a range of chemical-free essential oils with antifungal, antiseptic, and antibacterial properties to treat any kind of foot infection.

"What can I do about cracked heels?"

Rub Flexitol Heel Balm in twice a day and avoid sandals until your heels are smooth!

"Is there anything I can do about my chicken skin?"

Chicken skin (or keratosis pilaris) forms when protein buildups penetrate the hair follicle, causing small, acne-like bumps. Look for moisturizers containing propylene glycol to soften the skin, and lactic acid to help reduce the buildup of protein.

"Is waterproof mascara always best?"

Its ability to remain waterproof has its drawbacks: not only does it dry the lashes out, but people often end up stretching the skin and pulling lashes out in a bid to actually get it off again. Unless you're a regular swimmer, how many times do you find yourself face-up in a downpour or sobbing your mascara down your face?

"Are there any natural ingredients I should look for in an eye cream?"

Products that contain mallow are particularly useful. It's an anti-inflammatory that prevents lines and reduces puffiness.

"Which eye cream ingredients can banish dark circles?"

Seek out a product containing vitamin K to get rid of your dark circles, and alpha lipoic acid to brighten the skin.

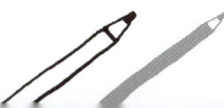

"Are there any miracle creams for under-eye shadows?"

Hylexin is the latest wonder cream to tackle these shadows, which, according to dermatologists, are caused by capillaries leaking blood and producing a dark, bruised look. Hylexin breaks down the pigmentation and reduces puffiness.

"How can I wake up with refreshed eyes?"

Look for the new beauty pads that are shaped to fit your under-eye area and contain ingredients such as caffeine to reduce puffiness, vitamin K to minimize dark circles, and vitamin C to fight wrinkles. Leave them on for the recommended time just before you go to bed.

"Can I increase the length of my eyelashes?"

New products, such as Lumigan, claim to boost lashes when applied daily for three months. They contain an active ingredient called bimatoprost.

"Will wearing lipstick every day do me any harm?"

Wearing lipstick can cause you to absorb up to 2 lb (1 kg) of potentially dangerous chemicals each year. Companies, such as the Green People in the UK, have formulated an organic lipstick, so learn from them and buy one that has natural colorings derived from earth minerals, not chemicals.

"Why isn't my lip balm curing my chapped lips?"

If it tastes nice, you may be licking your lips without realizing it and robbing them of yet more moisture. Look for balms containing beeswax, vitamin E, cocoa butter, or rice bran oil, plus sunscreen, of course.

"Are petroleum-based lip balms a cure or a curse?"

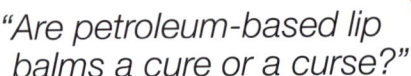

Petroleum acts as a plaster to the problem of dry lips, but doesn't actually cure the problem. Lips can also become "addicted" to petroleum balms, and so the more you use, the more you need to use. Better to stick to natural emollients such as almond, avocado, and coconut oils or shea butter.

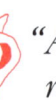

"Are there products that really reduce tooth sensitivity?"

Get hold of some specialist dentistry formula called Tooth Mousse, a water-based, sugar-free cream you rub onto your teeth twice a day to reduce hypersensitivity and prevent caries. Available in strawberry, vanilla, and melon flavor, it's even free of that nasty disinfectant taste of some dental products. Visit www.gcasia.info for more information.

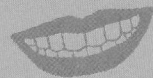

"How can I prevent tooth decay?"

Try finishing meals with a small amount of cheese. It is thought to protect tooth enamel by reducing acidity levels in the mouth.

"Is there anything I should look for with home teeth-bleaching kits?"

Make sure the pH reading is 7 or above. Anything lower will be too acidic and damage your teeth.

"What should a good toothpaste contain?"

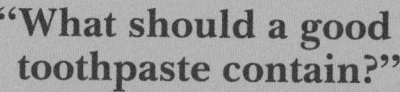

Look for sodium fluoride, sodium monofluorophosphate or a combination of the two, plus triclosan with either copolymer or zinc citrate for maximum plaque control and gum health.

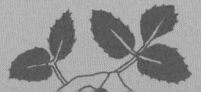

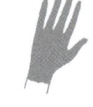

"I tend to get dry patches around my nails after painting them. What's the solution?"

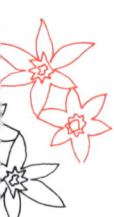

Formaldehyde, a chemical in most polishes, has been linked to everything from skin irritation to respiratory complaints, depression, and headaches and may even be carcinogenic. Zoya nail polishes (www.zoyapolish.co.uk) are free from formaldehyde and other potentially harmful chemicals.

"Which nail colors will suit me?"

For fair skin, choose berry reds and pale pinks with a blue undertone. For mid-tone skin, try dark and browny reds or caramel colors. For dark and black skins, opt for plums and berry colors, plus hot pinks and neons.

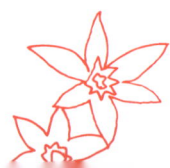

"Are quick-drying nail polishes best?"

If you're in a hurry, then a quick-drying polish is your only option. However, they're more prone to chipping, so make sure you apply a topcoat once a day when you have the time.

"Is perfume harmful to your skin?"

Fragrances are made almost entirely of chemicals. Nearly one-third of these are known to be toxic and may cause anything from allergies to cancer. Rub some essential oil or flower oil into your pulse points instead for chemical-free fragrance.

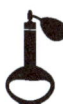

"How can I make my perfume go further?"

Solid perfumes have numerous advantages over liquid ones: they're often alcohol-free (so better for sensitive skins), they won't spill into the bottom of your handbag (what a waste) and the fragrance itself goes further and lasts longer.

"How do I find the perfect perfume?"

Follow your nose and the three golden rules: always test them on your skin, not on a taper; walk around the store for ten minutes to allow the scent to develop and mingle with your own body chemistry; buy different scents for different moods.

"Why does the smell of my perfume change from day to day?"

This is a real case of you are what you eat. Pungent foods like garlic can affect the body's chemistry and the way we smell, altering the scent of whichever perfume we apply.

"What's the best way to choose perfume?"

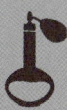

You need to understand the lingo of scent:

Floral is based on sweet flower fragrances, producing a very feminine smell.

Oriental combines deeper, musky fragrances, such as vanilla and exotic plants.

Woody can be deep, spicy, or burnt, with scents such as patchouli or even leather.

Water is light and refreshing. These scents may smell of air or a subtle sea breeze.

Citrus are oranges, lemons, and limes, often combined with other fruits for a zingy smell.

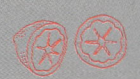

"Is it possible to go from brunette to blonde without using bleach?"

No. Highlighting of any sort requires a bleaching agent (usually hydrogen peroxide and ammonia) to remove pigment in the hair shaft.

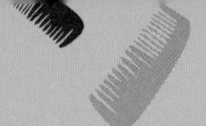

"How can I make my salon color last longer?"

If you find your hair (particularly gray strands) fading fast between salon appointments, use a color rinse shampoo that contains more gentle pigments to help keep your locks in a healthy condition.

"Are natural products better for my hair?"

As seductive as they sound, the words *natural*, *botanic,* and *herbal* count for very little. Any ingredient has to be preserved using chemicals, so the end product is completely different to the ingredient in its original form. Instead, look for products that are free from propylene glycol, PVP/VA copolymer, sodium laureth sulfate, parabens, flurocarbons, and synthetic colors and fragrances.

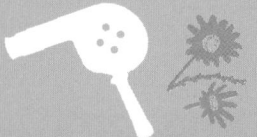

"How can I make my blow-dry last longer?"

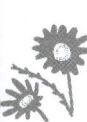

Hair aficionados have now developed dry shampoos: powders that you dust on to absorb grease from the roots and add volume for an extra day between washes.

"Which are the best hair straighteners to use?"

Telfon-coated irons that produce steam are best because they are less likely to dry the hair out.

"How often do I need to replace my hairbrush?"

Banish those tatty old combs and brushes with thinning bristles and get a new one once a year!

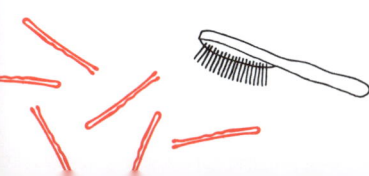

"How can I make my hairbrush last longer?"

Brushes with natural bristles will last the longest, and be kinder to your hair and scalp. Remember to clean your brush once a month by running a comb through the bristles to remove dead hair, oil, and bacteria.

"How can I give my hair more sheen?"

Just like the skin on your face, your scalp has a pH of between 4.5 and 5.5. Check that your shampoo and conditioner is neither lower (too acidic), nor higher (too alkaline), or look out for products that are *pH balanced*.

"How can I streamline my hair care regime?"

What with shampoos, conditioners, hair masks, sprays, and serums, hair can be a timely and costly business. Get a cheaper shampoo and splash out on a decent conditioner to use in the shower. Then use a leave-in conditioner to reduce frizz and create shine, so you don't need all the added extras.

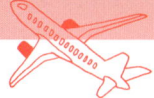

"How can I protect my hair from city pollution?"

Look out for shampoos with a UV filter and high antioxidant content to protect against free radical damage from the sun and city pollution.

"Is serum or wax better for taming my unruly hair?"

If stray flyaways are your problem, use a light serum, but avoid the roots or they'll look greasy. Coarse or curly hair is best treated with styling wax.

"Do I need to use a shampoo and conditioner from the same product range?"

This may seem like a scam, but products in the same range are made to complement one another and avoid adverse reactions. Make sure your shampoo and conditioner are targeted toward the same hair type, or you risk canceling out the benefits.

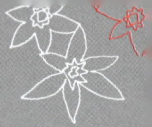

"How does vegetable dye differ from normal hair dye?"

Unlike permanent dyes, vegetable dyes contain no ammonia and are only temporary. They shampoo in, and offer a great starting point if you're experimenting with your color.

"What kind of shampoo will add volume to my hair?"

Look for shampoos containing dimethicone copolyol.

"My hair is flat at the roots and frizzy at the tips. Which products should I use?"

Combination hair, like combination skin, means different products for different areas. Use a volume-boosting mousse at the roots before blow-drying, then a smoothing serum on the tips afterward.

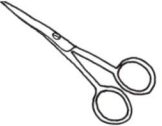

"Where can I find natural hair dye?"

Try Organic Color Systems and Tint of Nature, hair colorants that use natural ingredients, are free from ammonia, are not tested on animals and are made from ethical, sustainable resources. Visit www.organiccoloursystems.com for more information.

"How is a clarifying shampoo different from a normal one?"

Clarifying shampoos are stronger and have a higher pH (are more alkaline). They remove a buildup of products, hard water, or chlorine from your hair.

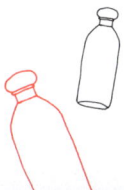

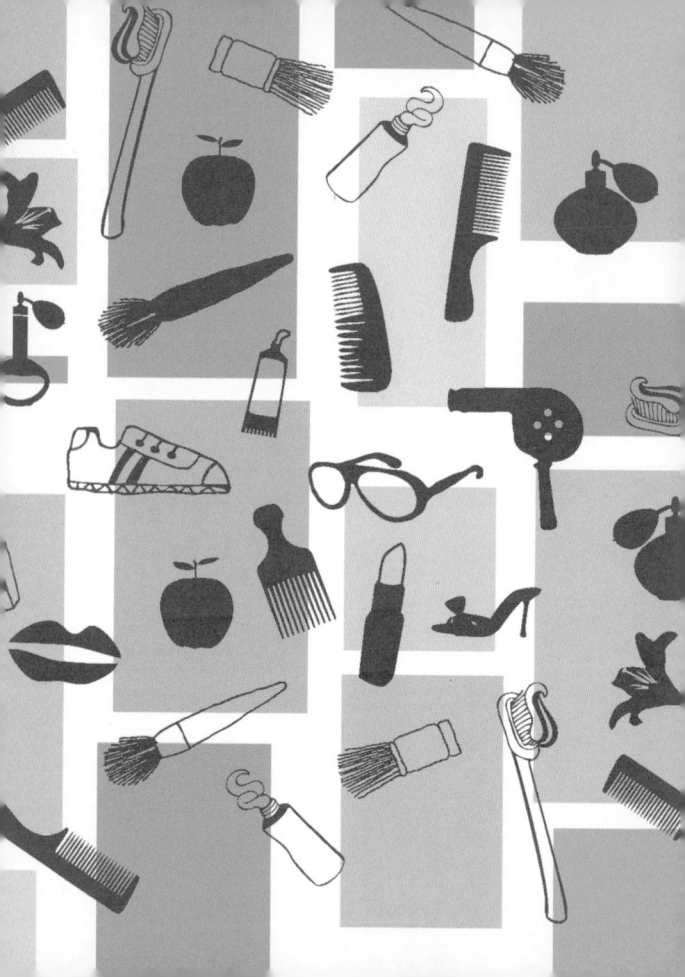

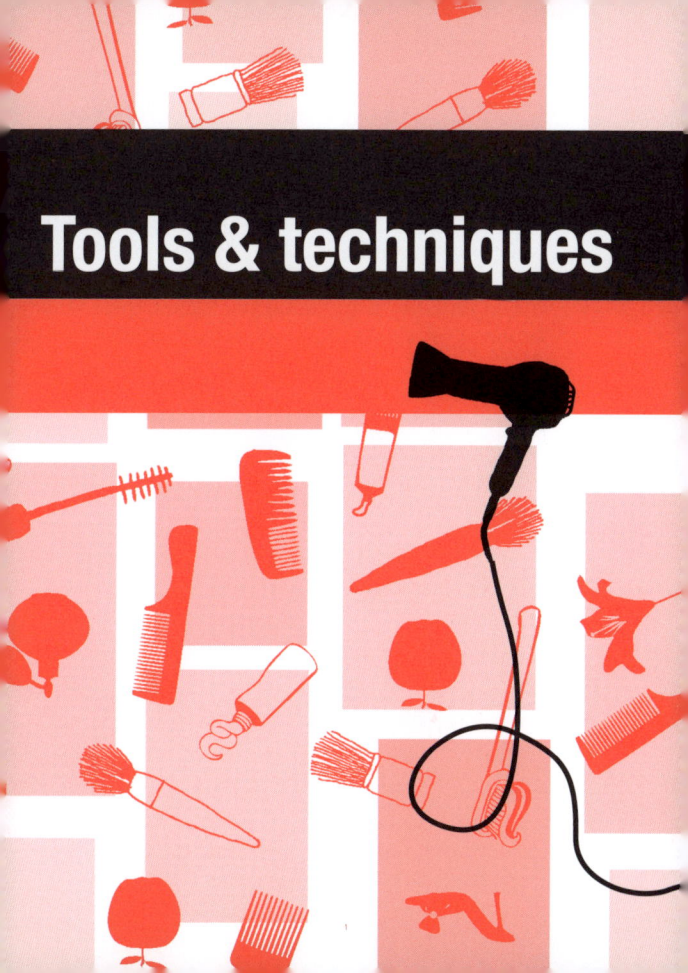
Tools & techniques

"When applying make-up, which brushes do I use for each product?"

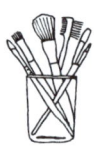

Use a sponge for foundation, nylon brushes for cream and liquid products, and large brushes for powders. In general, the softer the bristles, the more natural and even the look. Firmer brushes provide a more solid application.

"What's the best way to apply foundation to cover large pores?"

Ditch the sponge and dab on small amounts with your finger before blending. Applying with a brush or sponge can make it go on too thickly, clogging your pores even more.

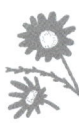

"What do I need to make my pores seem smaller?"

Arm yourself with a microfiber facecloth and use it to cleanse your face twice a day. The gently exfoliating action will help draw out the impurities that make your pores look large.

"How can I stop my lip gloss from looking gloopy?"

Apply it with a small brush, rather than straight from the tube, to get an even coverage and less gloop.

"Do I really need to use toner?"

Toner restores the skin to its natural pH after cleansing, keeping its protective barrier intact. Repeat the mantra: cleanse, tone, moisturize.

"What's the best way to cleanse my face?"

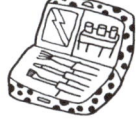

Use the pads of your fingertips in small circular movements to massage the cleanser into your skin and boost circulation. Leave it on for a few minutes so it has time to work thoroughly before rinsing.

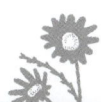

"What's the best way to apply moisturizer?"

Always apply in long, upward-sweeping movements. Never neglect your neck and never use a downward motion as it'll drag your skin down too.

"How can I exfoliate in a gentle way?"

If your skin is sensitive to abrasive exfoliators, use a muslin cloth instead; the texture of the fabric gently removes dead skin cells. Wash the cloth regularly so it doesn't harbor bacteria.

"What else can I do for my skin at home?"

Give yourself regular facial massages, using small circular movements in an upward direction to relax the muscles, improve circulation, and soften fine lines.

"Why won't my foundation go on smoothly?"

If you've already exfoliated and moisturized before applying your foundation, facial hair could be the problem. If you suffer from excess hair, get it threaded to stop your foundation caking on the hairs and making them look more obvious.

"How can I depuff my face in the morning?"

When you put on your moisturizer, take three or four minutes to give your face a massage, paying particular attention to the area around the eyes, to disperse excess fluid.

"How can I wake up with smooth skin on my face?"

Add a dollop of an alpha hydroxy acid exfoliator to your usual nighttime moisturizer. It'll set to work on those dead skin cells while you get your beauty sleep.

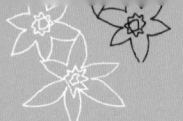

"What's the best technique for all-over great skin?"

Give yourself a prebedtime checklist: face cream, eye cream, lip balm, hand cream.

"What's the best way to body brush?"

Body brushing is said to stimulate blood flow to the skin, exfoliate away dead skin cells, and encourage new cell growth. Buy a natural brush with soft bristles that won't scratch the skin. Brush in circular movements, sweeping up from your feet toward the heart. Use a long-handled brush for your back.

"How can I stop myself from falling out of my low-cut dress?"

Avoid embarrassing mishaps by carrying a few strips of Hollywood fashion tape. It's double-sided and will adhere to both skin and fabric so you can stick yourself into your dress and dance the night away without worrying.

"How can I stop my bed sheets from getting stained after I apply fake tan?"

For anyone with a sense of humor, the Tangro jumpsuit is like a giant pink onesie that you sleep in after self-tanning. Not to be attempted when you've got company.

"How can I keep my elbows and knees streak-free when self-tanning?"

Streakiness and a general look of grubbiness occur because the skin is usually drier and more uneven in these places. After exfoliating well, apply some olive oil over the rough patches to help the tan glide on more smoothly.

"How can I stop fake tan from collecting in my creases?"

Always stretch the skin out and apply tan to bent knees and elbows where there tend to be more natural creases.

"How can I hide the telltale fake tan signs?"

Wash your hands immediately after using a fake tan product and swipe a face cleansing wipe over your brow, along your hairline, over your ankles and in the creases of your elbows and knees.

"What can I do about my cellulite?"

Try a finger-pinching massage using your thumb and forefinger to gently stimulate blood flow to the area and help reduce the buildup of fatty tissue.

"How can I get all-over silky-smooth skin?"

When exfoliating and body brushing, pay particular attention to the elbows, knees, thighs, and buttocks where rough patches or cellulite have a tendency to form.

"If a little antiaging cream is good for me, is a lot even better?"

Putting a double dose of cream on won't wipe away double the number of wrinkles. Always follow the dosages on your cosmetics bottles to avoid buildup and skin sensitivity or allergies.

"How can I stop my hands from aging?"

While most of us have realized the importance of using a sunscreen on our faces, we often forget our hands. When you're done with your face, just wipe the excess on the backs of your hands to give them the protection they need.

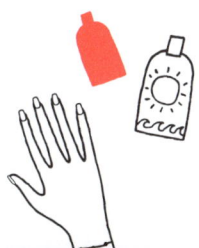

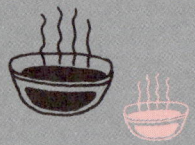

"Is there a right way to squeeze pimples?"

Popping generally causes the infection to spread. If you really can't help yourself, wash your hands, steam your face over a pan of hot water for a few minutes and wrap your forefingers in tissue before applying gentle pressure. Never use your nails because you'll damage the skin.

"What techniques can I use to avoid breakouts?"

If you apply your concealer and foundation with a brush or sponge, make sure you wash them between each use or you risk spreading the bacteria around your face.

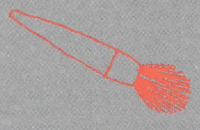

"How can I unblock my pores and resist the urge to squeeze them?"

Get into steaming. Cover your head with a towel and lean over a bowl of boiling water for five minutes or so to open the pores. Cleanse with a gentle cleanser, then splash with cold water to close the pores again. Better still, invest in a professional steamer.

"How can I prevent hairline breakouts?"

This could be a reaction to styling products on your hair. Stick to products that you apply with your hands (not sprays), and keep them well away from your skin.

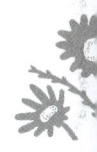

"Are there gadgets to zap away pimples?"

New gizmos, such as Spot Treatment by Zeno, heat up to just the right temperature to destroy bacteria without damaging the skin. You apply the gadget to the pimple, wait for it to do its magic, and expect to see a clearer complexion soon after.

"Can I recreate salon treatments at home?"

The latest gadgets allow you to get the treatment without the price tag. Tools such as the Roc Renew Microdermabrasion System come with a grainy scrub and a battery-operated applicator to give a salonlike exfoliation.

"Are there any gadgets for instant facial toning?"

Nu Face is a hand-held gizmo that delivers microcurrents to the skin to stimulate muscle contractions and tighten the face.

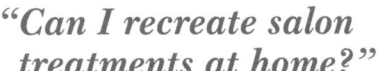

"What beauty gadgets do the celebs use?"

Oprah is reportedly a fan of the Clarisonic Cleansing Brush. It's battery-operated, uses two oscillating brushes and claims to remove more make-up than normal fingertip cleansing.

"Should I shave or exfoliate first?"

Gentle exfoliation helps prepare the skin and can help you get a closer shave.

"Is it okay to shave with soap?"

Soap usually has a drying effect on the skin, so does not act as a good lubricant when shaving. Choose foams and gels that contain cooling ingredients such as aloe vera to soothe, rather than irritate, the skin.

"How can I prevent ingrown hairs after shaving?"

These are caused when hairs grow back on themselves and penetrate the skin, causing redness, tenderness, and swelling. To prevent them, use a moisture-rich shaving cream, shave less frequently, and always in the direction of hair growth. Avoid using the razor repeatedly over the same area.

"How can I make my perfume last longer?"

Fragrances tend to evaporate more quickly from the surface of dry skin so apply a layer of moisturizer before your scent to keep it there for longer.

"How can I smell heavenly all day long?"

Learn how to layer your scent. Start with some eau de toilette, then add a few drops of perfume on your hair and pulse points, and finish by applying a body cream that matches your perfume.

"How can I give my eyes an instant lift?"

Get yourself an Eye Pen and Serum kit. The wandlike gadget creates a pulsating action that forces the active ingredients of the serum to penetrate deeper into the skin. It plumps and tightens the muscles around the eyes in an instant.

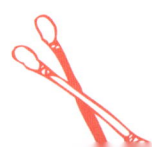

> "How can I stop my eyes from feeling gritty first thing in the morning?"

This might be caused by eye products becoming trapped in the eye overnight. Always apply eye creams and serums to the bone just below the eye in a semicircle up to the brow bone and never take it right up to the lash line.

"I've overplucked my eyebrows. How can I get them back on track?"

The fashion for matchstick-thin brows has been replaced by fuller, more defined ones. Rub castor oil on your brows once a day to encourage regrowth, then forbid yourself to touch them until they look scraggy and over-grown. Book yourself a once-monthly appointment for threading, plucking, or waxing, and don't be tempted to perform touchups in between. The cultivation period is tiresome, but it'll be worth it.

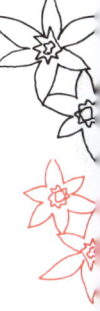

"How do I get the perfect eyebrow shape?"

Good brows can act like a natural facelift. When plucking, ensure the highest point of the arch falls at the outer third of the eye as you go toward your ears. The brow should follow the natural curve of the eye, beginning at the corner and not overextending into the temple.

"Should I keep my brows full or create a thinner arch?"

Like everything, brow shapes come and go. You can create more of an arch by creating a thinner line of hair, but plucking them to within an inch of their lives is incredibly aging. We naturally lose hair (brows included) as we age, so keep hold of whatever you have and just keep them tidy with regular salon appointments.

"When's the best time to pluck my eyebrows?"

After a bath or shower when the skin is more supple and the pores have been opened. Avoid plucking during the week before your period when your skin is more sensitive.

"How can I keep my nail polish chip-free for longer?"

Follow the five golden rules:

- Invest in a good-quality nail polish; salon brands such as Essie, OPI and Jessica are best.
- Always apply a base coat before the color and a topcoat afterward.
- Make sure nails are dry between coats.
- Paint right up to and over the ends of your nails.
- Apply a fresh layer of topcoat each day.

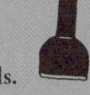
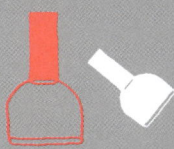

"What's the best way to shape your nails?"

A standard question in nail salons is, "square or round?" The answer nowadays is squoval, (square-oval). Whichever you choose, don't round the edges. Squaring the corners increases strength and minimizes the risk of an in-grown nail.

"How can I get perfectly finished nails using a dark polish?"

When using dark colors, leave a thin strip at the sides of your nails because the polish tends to bleed a little before setting.

"How can I stop my nails from splitting when I file them?"

Sweep the file (a glass one if possible) in one direction only instead of sawing backward and forward.

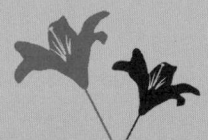

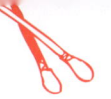

"How can I clean the dirt from under my nails?"

Dip the end of a toothpick in some nail polish remover and lightly roll it in a cotton ball. This will make a cotton swab that is narrower than a regular one so it can squeeze right under the nails.

"How can I get my nail polish smooth?"

Instead of shaking the bottle before you apply, roll it between your hands to warm the liquid and prevent air bubbles from forming.

"How can I make my nails look longer?"

Leave a gap at the side of your nails when painting them to make them appear longer and thinner.

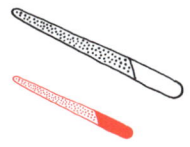

"Do I really have to floss as well as brush my teeth?"

Cleaning your teeth is like having a good manicure (well almost). After you've buffed and filed your nails, you wouldn't leave all that dirt underneath them would you? After you've brushed your teeth, flossing removes plaque from the surfaces of the tooth and gum that the brush can't reach, protecting you from gum disease.

"What's the best way to floss my teeth?"

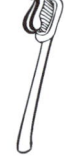

Instead of using a sawing action, wrap the floss around the base of the tooth and gently pull it upward to remove lodged food particles.

"How often should I wash my hair?"

If you can get away with every other day, do so. Consider washing it less in the winter when the air is drier and central heating works to sap your hair of moisture.

"I wash my hair frequently but it still looks dull. Why is that?"

A common cause of dull hair is insufficient rinsing. Use a small amount of shampoo, massage it into your scalp for 30 seconds, then rinse and rinse again twice.

"What's the best way to wash your hair?"

Use the smallest amount of shampoo you can get away with and make time to give yourself a slow scalp massage to boost circulation and clean it thoroughly. Comb a conditioner through and leave for two minutes, then rinse, rinse, and rinse again.

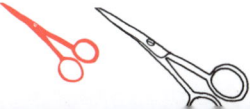

"Do I have to condition my hair?"

The trick with hair washing is quality, not quantity. Always use a small amount of shampoo and rinse well, trying not to tangle your hair. Long, thick, and dry hair may need conditioning at every wash, but fine hair may only need a mild conditioner once a week. Avoid applying to the roots unless your scalp is very dry because this will make them go flat.

"Is it necessary to shampoo twice in one wash?"

Some experts say that two washes are needed to clean the hair properly, but unless you've been camping, it's unlikely that your locks will be that filthy. Stick to one shampoo and prevent stripping away the scalp's natural oils needed for healthy hair.

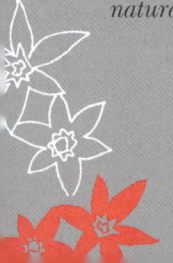
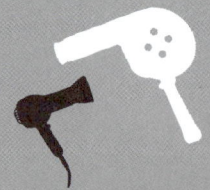

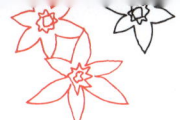

"How can I make the most of expensive hair masks?"

If you've splashed out, you'll want to get your money's worth. Always apply the mask and wrap a towel around your head (if it's been heated up first, even better) to allow the ingredients to penetrate more deeply.

"What is hair build-up?"

This is when ingredients in the products you use literally build up, leaving your hair dull and prone to undesirable color changes. Look for special detoxing products, which are left on for a few minutes and are designed to remove this excess.

"Will leaving my hair partially wet damage it?"

On the contrary, blow-drying your hair until it's completely dry will leave it prone to breakages. Go to 80 percent dry, then let the air do the rest naturally.

"How can I tame my curly hair?"

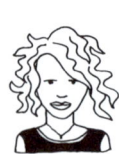

Never wring it dry or rub at it with a towel—you'll only increase the frizz. Blot it gently between sheets of paper towel to dry it, then use moisturizing and smoothing products before styling.

"What's the best way to brush hair without causing breakages?"

Choose a brush with widely spaced plastic bristles and work from the tips up.

"What's the best brush to use on wet hair?"

Use a vented brush with slats down the middle that won't trap the moisture.

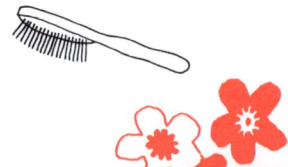

TOOLS & TECHNIQUES

"How can I tame my flyaway baby hair?"

Spray a little hairspray onto an old toothbrush and use it to tame those pesky strays beside your face.

"How can I make my hair look sleek and glossy but not greasy?"

Steer clear of oil-based products, such as serums and mousses, and use hairspray, which is naturally drier. Spray some into your palms, rub them together and smooth over from just below the roots to the tips.

"How do I prevent bed-head?"

If you generally wake up looking like you've spent the night with your finger in an electric outlet, sleep on a silk pillowcase to stop your hair from snagging and tangling.

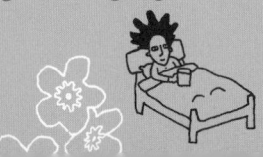

"What's the best way to blow-dry bangs?"

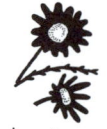

Stop it from falling flat by brushing and drying to one side, then the other, then letting it rest in the middle.

"How can I minimize the damage to my hair from styling tools?"

Always use a heat-protecting spray and keep your dryer, curling iron, or straighteners moving, rather than frazzling one section under the heat for a few seconds.

"How can I get beachy waves in my hair?"

Try tying your hair in a low ponytail and wetting it under a running faucet. Wring it out, then untie it when it's dry for soft, surfer-girl curls.

"What's the best brush to use for blow-drying hair smooth?"

If you want silky smooth locks, use a round brush to wind the hair around and pull the hair gently downward.

"How can I make my hair-styling tools last longer?"

Just like emptying a vacuum cleaner full of debris to keep it in working order, you need to rid your styling tools of any styling products and stray hair. Wipe curling irons and straighteners down after each use (wait for them to cool down first) and check the inside of your hairdryer for hair after every few uses.

"How can I detangle my unruly hair?"

The Tangle Teezer is a new form of brush invented by a celebrity colorist. It claims to be able to undo even the trickiest knots in wet or dry hair without causing breakages.

"How can I blow-dry my flyaway hair smooth?"

Use an ionic drier, which releases a stream of charged ions to surround the hair and help prevent a buildup of static.

"How can I get a smooth finish on my long hair?"

After blow-drying, use a small amount of smoothing serum on the ends and finish it by brushing with a paddle brush.

TOOLS & TECHNIQUES

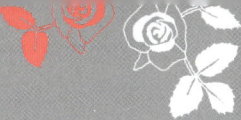

"How can I add body to super-fine hair?"

Use large, heated curlers for big curls with volume. Apply a heat-protecting spray before and a light hairspray afterward to stop them from dropping out.

"How can I get better curls when I'm blow-drying my hair?"

Spray hairspray onto your brush before you curl the hair around it to give it extra bounce and hold.

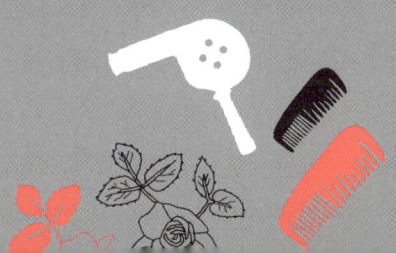

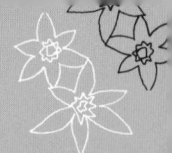

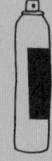

"How can I make my hair less flyaway after blow-drying?"

Always blow-dry with the nozzle facing downward and move along the hair from root to tip. This helps the hair cuticle lie flat, making your hair look sleeker.

"How can I get the crimped hair look that I've seen on the catwalks?"

This is not the hit-and-miss affair of your childhood experiments: catwalk crimping is neat, sleek, and even. To get the look, dry your hair straight, apply a heatproof spray, then swipe professional crimpers down the hair from root to tip. Leave it loose or tie a half-head section up at the back.

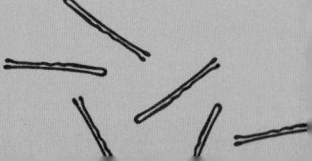

"What's the best way to grow out a bad haircut?"

Although it might be tempting never to let a pair of scissors within arm's reach of your locks again, resist this urge. Keep up your regular appointments, trimming split ends and reshaping your style as it grows longer.

"What's the best way to grow out highlights?"

It can be tempting to try dying your hair back to its natural color, but this rarely gives a convincing effect and can give your highlights a greenish tinge. Ask your colorist to begin adding lowlights each time you visit and gradually make your hair darker as the highlights grow out.

"Does perfume go off?"

Although perfumes come without a "best before" date, they can sometimes deteriorate long before you have finished the bottle. Perfume that hasn't been stored correctly is likely to race past its prime—its scent starts to smell sour and the colour turns darker. To make a perfume last longer keep it away from direct light and heat.

"What are the best products to use with hair extensions?"

Hair extensions require dedicated upkeep to remain looking luscious. Conditioning products containing a cocktail of vitamins and proteins will revitalize and preserve, while shampoo containing Pro-vitamin B5 will cleanse and nourish hair and protect bonds. It is important to consult your hair stylist on the compatibility of any products you are not sure of, because some products can loosen braids.

"Should you apply concealer over or under foundation?"

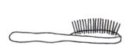

If you are trying to cover a blemish then foundation comes first and concealer is dabbed on afterward. If you are covering dark under eye circles use concealer only and keep foundation away from this delicate area.

"Do I need to swap shampoo with the seasons?"

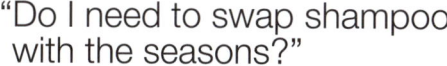

In the summer your hair has to defend itself against more enemies, such as the sun, sea salt, excess sweat, and chlorine, so switching to a gentler shampoo can help to keep your hair soft without stripping it of its natural oils.

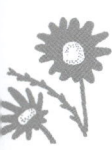

"What should I use to cover my tattoo in an emergency?"

Try Dermablend®, a dense foundation that lasts for hours and can be used on the body.

"How can I transform my office make-up into an instant party look?"

If you've only got five minutes for a transformation, don't waste time by removing your day make-up. Instead, use it as a smooth base. Mix your foundation with a light primer and smooth over your face to revive your skin, then work on with dramatic eyes or bold lips, not both. A dab of blush on the apples of your cheeks and some highlighter swept above your cheekbones and below your brows will finish your look. Clean your teeth, spritz on perfume, and don't even think about polishing your nails.

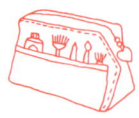

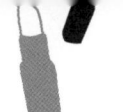

"Should I apply my day make-up and night make-up in different ways?"

Always have light falling evenly on your face when applying make-up: during the day use natural light from a window, if possible, at night use a mirror with bulbs fixed all around it. For daytime, warm the skin with a yellowish (rather than blue) base and a bronzer close to your own skin tone. Don't go too heavy on the powder—harsh light will make you look caked. For candlelit evenings you can afford to go a bit darker with the bronzer (just avoid an obvious line around the jaw) and beef up your lips or eyes with more color.

"How can I streamline my make-up bag?"

If you don't want to cart around half your body weight in make-up, opt for multitasking products that can be used on eyes, lips, and cheeks. Products such as The Multiple by Nars (www.narscosmetics.co.uk) work as a blush, highlighter, and add a shimmer to the lips, all in one compact stick.

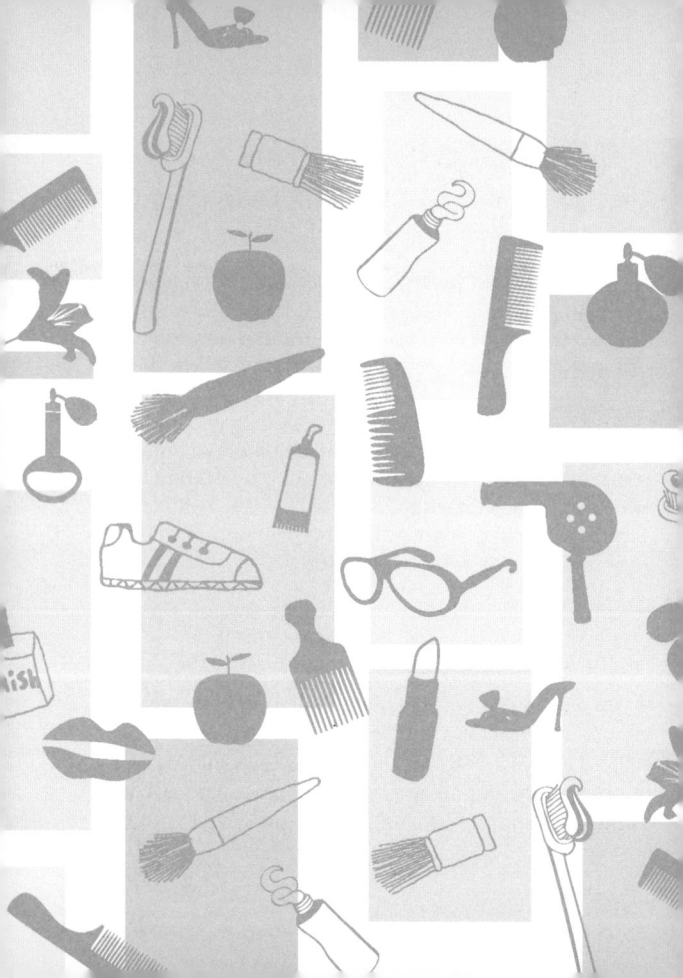

Applying make-up

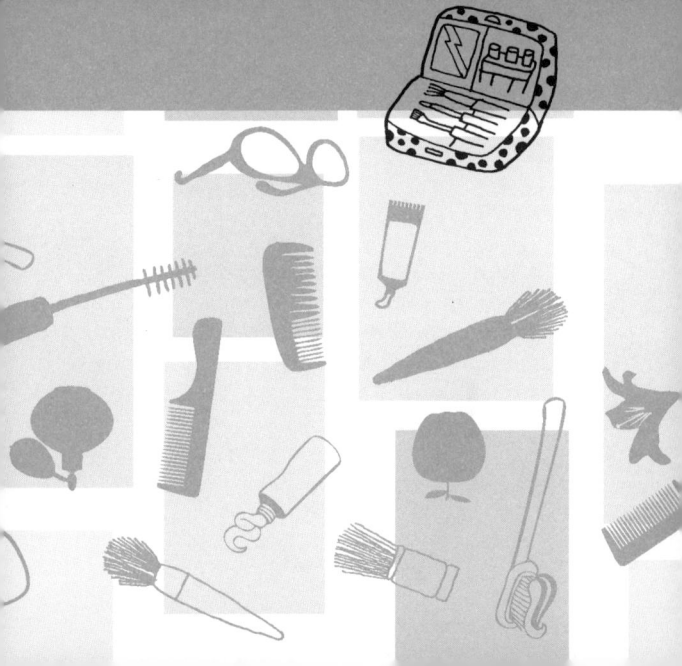

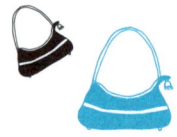

"How can I be more adventurous with my make-up?"

First, accept that most of us can only wear colors within a fairly narrow spectrum. The trick is to find which shades flatter you, be they browns, pinks, or apricots, and then experiment with new products within this range when you feel like a change.

"Glitter or no glitter?"

Unless you're going to a costume party, leave the glitter firmly alone. Iridescent eye shadows and mixing a small amount of shimmer with your foundation will add a subtle glow.

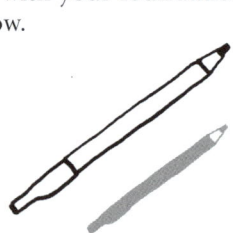

"How can I get a flawless complexion with make-up?"

Preparation is the key. After you've moisturized, prepare the skin with a primer to smooth and brighten your skin. Dot an oil-free liquid foundation on areas where there is discoloration (blemishes, broken veins, under-eye shadows, and the inner corner of the eye), then pat in gently with fingers or a damp cosmetic sponge. Paint an extra layer of lighter-colored concealer under the eyes using a make-up brush. Apply a light dusting of loose powder with a large brush to set and seal your flawless complexion.

"What's a fail-safe way to find my perfect foundation?"

It's pointless to test foundation on your hand, which is usually darker than the skin on your face. Instead, dab it onto your jawline. The right shade will look as if it has disappeared.

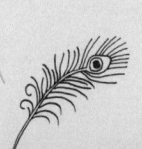

"How can I make my foundation last longer?"

If you're frugal with your foundation, it can spoil before you've finished the bottle. Always buy foundation in bottles with a pump to help keep bacteria out and maximize its shelf life.

"How do I find the right concealer for me?"

Using the wrong shade will highlight rather than hide your flaws, so follow the basic rules: Concealer with a greenish tinge will hide redness; a blue tone will complement fair skin; a yellow concealer is good for dark or uneven skin; while a pinkish color will illuminate a dull complexion.

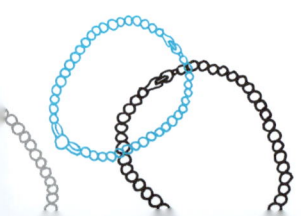

"How do I get a winter glow?"

Bronzer is supposed to warm, not color, the skin so buy one that is close to your natural skin tone. Use a large, soft-bristled brush to sweep it over the parts where the sun naturally hits: cheeks, forehead, chin, and the bridge of your nose. Follow with a dusting of warm, pinkish blush on the apples of the cheeks.

"Can I test the color of a new foundation over my make-up?"

Never test foundations over any make-up you already have on. However, if you can't face the trauma of going bare-faced into a shop, do a small test on the inside of your arm to find the nearest shade.

"When it comes to skin, is matt always better?"

Not necessarily. To get the fresh-faced, dewy look that is popular at the moment, try a foundation or concealer with light-reflecting pigments. It's particularly flattering on older skins and will stop you from looking caked.

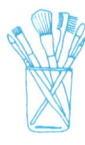

"How can I avoid a caked look when applying foundation?"

Other than choosing a lighter formula, use a latex sponge (dampening it slightly first) to apply and get a more sheer coverage.

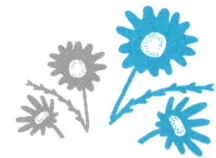

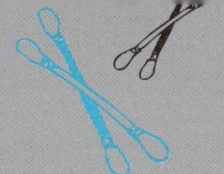

"I'm pale but not interesting. How can I get a healthy glow?"

Remember the rule: if you don't want to end up looking grubby, bronzers should never be two shades darker than your skin tone. Facial tanning products often block pores, leaving blackheads more visible, so your best bet is a light tinted moisturizer (with an SPF if possible). Apply this as your base then dust a light layer of rose or gold bronzer on your cheekbones, chin, and down your nose where the sun would naturally hit your face.

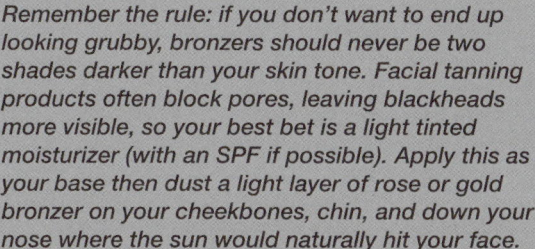

"Where should I apply highlighter?"

Under your eyebrows, down the middle of your nose, just above your cupid's bow, and in a semicircle from your outer eye along the line of your cheekbone. Avoid blemishes at all costs because you don't want to highlight them too.

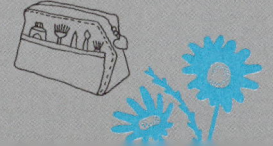

"What's the key to buying products for the natural look?"

Look for words such as "tint" (on products that provide a sheer coverage) and "illuminating" (on products that contain light-reflecting particles) to give you a fresh-faced, dewy look.

"What should I look for when buying make-up for oily skin?"

Avoid anything labeled "illuminating," because this will only add shine to your face. Instead, seek products with the words "mattifying", "cream to powder," or "long lasting" on the label. All of them will combat shine and cling to your skin all day.

"What's the perfect consistency for concealer?"

Under-eye concealer should be light and creamy (it smoothes out a long way when you try it on your hand). For acne, it should be thick and pasty to stick to the skin, rather than glide along it.

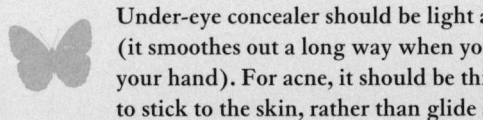

"None of the foundations I've tried suits me. How do I find one that does?"

Cosmetics companies, such as Prescriptives, now offer a customized service to match foundation to your skin tone.

"Can I hide my wrinkles with foundation?"

Foundation tends to sit in, rather than cover up, cracks making your lines look all the more obvious. Instead, opt for a tinted moisturizer or primer with light-reflecting particles to give you a youthful glow.

"Should I apply foundation or concealer first?"

Use a thin layer of foundation only on the areas that are patchy or uneven, then apply a thicker concealer to provide a double coating over bigger blemishes.

"What color foundation suits Asian skin tones?"

Choose a foundation with a yellow undertone to enhance, rather than work against, your natural coloring.

"What's the best way of covering the darker areas on my face?"

When applying concealer, place a lamp above your face to bring out the shadows (where you need most coverage) and show you the places to highlight, those where the light falls naturally.

"How can I get a contoured effect without complicated shading?"

Overzealous shading can leave you looking grubby rather than glowy. To give your face an extra kick, blend some liquid highlighter with your usual foundation or a gel blush and apply as normal. It'll catch the light in all the right areas.

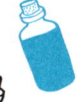

"What type of foundation is best for dark skin?"

Dark skins tend to be oilier so use a cream- or powder-based foundation to balance out the shine.

"How can I get a healthy-looking flush?"

If you have a tendency to overdo the blush, keep two brushes for applying your rouge. Use one to sweep it over the apples of your cheeks, and keep the other one clean to buff over the top afterward to remove any excess and ensure it's properly blended.

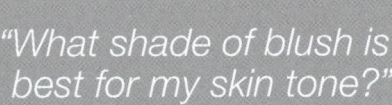

"What shade of blush is best for my skin tone?"

Very pale skin tones: stick to pale pinks, apricots, and beiges. Anything stronger will overpower your face.

Yellowish skins: counterbalance your natural tone with warmer coral tones.

Pinkish skins: minimize red tones, which will highlight your natural tone; opt instead for a contrasting apricot.

Olive skins: go for pinks or peaches with a gold undertone.

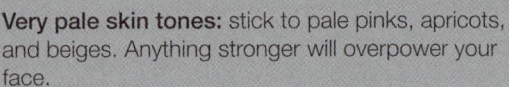

"Which shades of blush will work on my dark skin?"

Accentuate the natural warmth in your skin by choosing dusty pink and copper tones with an undertone of gold for the evening.

"How do I know which color blush will suit me best?"

Try matching the color to the one that appears naturally when you pinch your cheeks.

"Do cream or powder blushes give a better effect?"

Cream blushes give a wonderfully smooth, dewy effect on normal skin. However, if your skin is oily, it can add to the shine so stick to an oil-fee version of traditional powder.

"What's the best way to accentuate my cheekbones?"

Apply blush on the apples of your cheeks only, sweep bronzer just below this, then dot highlighter in a semi-circle along your cheekbones and up to your brows.

"How can I disguise my ruddy cheeks?"

If you suffer from rosacea, use a foundation with a green undertone to help balance out your flushed complexion.

"What are the rules when it comes to shading?"

Repeat the mantra: anything you make darker will recede, anything you make lighter will be brought forward.

"How can I bring out the blue in my eyes?"

Switch from black mascara and eyeliner to brown or violet shades. They'll also make the whites of your eyes look whiter.

"How can I make my eyes look bigger?"

After you've blended eye shadow over the lids, put a dot of very light, iridescent shadow in the very middle. This will open up the eyes and stop darker shading from making your eyes look smaller.

"How can I make my eyes look brighter?"

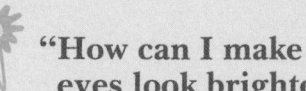

Instead of using your usual black eyeliner and mascara, choose cobalt blue or gray products.

"How can I make my eyes look farther apart?"

It's all about light and dark. Dot a pale concealer in the inner corners of your eyes and use a darker shadow or liner at the outer corners.

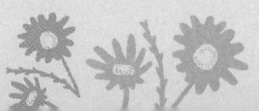

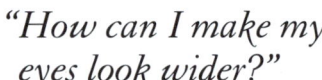

"How can I make my eyes look wider?"

Use a shadow as close to the natural color of your eyelids as possible and blend all the way up to the brow bone. Don't forget to dot some in the inner corners of your eyes.

"What's the best way to conceal the bags under my eyes?"

Using a brush, apply concealer liberally and leave it to set slightly for a couple of minutes. Pat in with your fingertips then sweep the excess color upward with a brush to stop it from sitting in lines and exaggerating any wrinkles. Never forget to dab a small spot in the corner of your eyes for a youthful appearance.

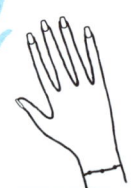

"How much concealer should I apply to hide my under-eye circles?"

Less is always more. Start by dabbing on a very thin layer using your middle finger, wait for it to dry, then build up another layer if necessary. Never just *slap* it all on at once—it'll only sit in the creases.

"How do I stop my mascara from clumping?"

Never pump the wand in the container. As air gets inside, it dries the liquid, leaving you with clogged lashes.

"What's the best way to apply mascara?"

Wipe away any clumps on the wand, then start at the roots of your lashes, moving the wand from side to side as you progress toward the tips. This way you'll ensure even coverage and separate your lashes at the same time.

"How can I stop my mascara from flaking and smudging?"

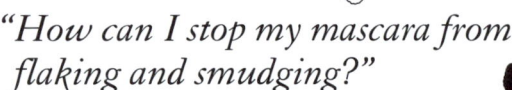

The filaments in many lengthening and volumizing mascaras can lead to smudging. Ask at the beauty counter for one that is free from filaments.

"What type of mascara wand is easiest to use?"

It depends on the look you are trying to achieve. For volume, use straight, solid wands to deposit more mascara onto the lashes, especially at the base. For lengthening, choose closely packed, soft bristles to apply a thinner coat that sweeps up the curve of the lash. For speed, a curved wand will follow the natural shape of the eye and coat all the lashes in one go.

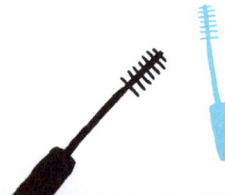

"Is there a way to make my mascara last longer?"

Lightly dust some loose powder over your lashes before applying mascara.

"How can I create a smudgy look with my eyeliner?"

Allow your kohl pencil to sit in some warm water for a while before applying it.

"How can I get my liquid eyeliner smooth and even?"

Pros can do it in one quick lick of the wand, but if your hands are little shaky, place a few evenly spaced dots along the lash line for guidance, then go back and join them up afterward.

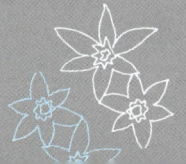

"How can I stop my kohl from breaking?"

Put it in the freezer for 15 minutes before applying it and always sharpen it after each use.

"How can I stop my eyeliner from smudging?"

Set your liner by applying some powder in the same color over the top.

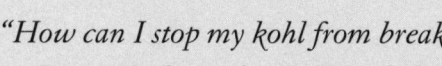

"Why does eyeliner always look so severe?"

Many eyeliners, particularly liquid ones, give a solid, severe effect. Soften your look by wetting a thin brush and using some brown eye shadow as a liner instead.

"Which eye shadow colors suit Asian skin tones?"

Go for smudgy grays and sheer, pale shades.

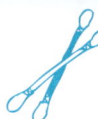

"How can I make my eye make-up last longer?"

Smooth a lightly colored foundation or concealer over your lids before applying your eye shadow.

"Which eye shadow colors will suit me best?"

Make-up artists generally agree that contrasting colors are best. For blue eyes, choose brown or lavender shadows; for brown eyes, choose green or blue; for green eyes, burnt oranges or browns work best. Neutral and gold shadows generally work on all eye colors.

"Which eye shadow colors work best on dark skins?"

For an understated look, choose deep burgundies, plums and coppers to complement your warm skin tone. If you're feeling more adventurous, you have one of the few skin tones that can take neon brights such as electric blue or apple green.

"What are the best products for making my eyes **pop***?"*

Avoid hard lines and solid edges from liquid liners and instead blend, blend, blend three shades of shadow that complement each other, working the darkest one into the outer corner of the eye and natural crease.

"How can I get my false eye lashes to look more natural?"

Avoid looking like a man in drag by trimming the corner lashes with (clean) nail scissors to even the lash set out.

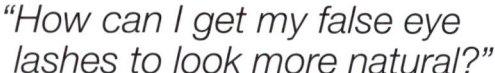

"Can I create a subtle effect with false lashes?"

Cut each set in half and apply the lashes only to the corners of your eyes for a more subtle, fluttery effect.

"What's the secret to making smoky eyes?"

- *Prep the eyelid with some foundation or a primer.*
- *Apply a neutral shadow all over the eyelid up to the brow.*
- *Use a kohl liner to line the upper lashes, making the line thicker in the middle.*
- *Do the same on the bottom, then use your finger to smudge the line.*
- *Apply shadow on the top to set the liner.*
- *Use a clean brush to smudge the shadow at the outer corner of the eye and work it into the lid's natural crease.*
- *Put a dot of shimmery shadow in the middle of the lid and in the inner corner.*
- *Finish with two coats of mascara.*

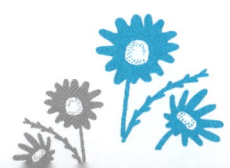

"How do I pick the right eyebrow pencil?"

The wrong shade can make you look alarmingly scary, so follow this guide:

Black brows: use a soft black or dark gray pencil.

Dark brown brows: choose a mahogany brown.

Mid-brown brows: go for chocolate.

Dark blonde brows: fawns are best; if you have a natural reddish tint choose caramel.

Blonde brows: ash or taupe; avoid anything too yellow or light because eyebrows are naturally darker than the hair on your head.

"What's the best way to conceal overplucked brows?"

Use a brow pencil to lightly fill in the gaps. When choosing a shade, err on the side of caution and never go darker than your natural brow color.

"Gloss or lipstick?"

If you want high shine, pick gloss. If it's bold color you want, choose lipstick. Tinted lip balm is a halfway house, but high gloss and strong color is way too much.

"How can I make my lipstick last longer?"

With all the talking, eating, drinking, and kissing our mouths do, no lipstick is ever going to be infallible. Dab concealer on your lips before applying your lipstick for some damage limitation.

"When it comes to lipstick, is liner or no liner best?"

Lip liner can help define your lips and stop your lipstick from bleeding. Pick a shade close to your natural lip color so when your lipstick fades, you're not left looking like a clown with an overly dark outline.

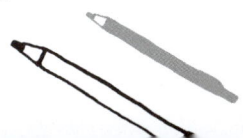

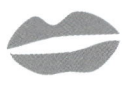

"What's the best way to even out my lipstick?"

Spread your lips into a gentle smile and never pucker.

"How can I make the nude lips look work?"

Pale skins should pick peaches, pinks, and even the palest of beiges, while olive tones must opt for warmer shades with brown. Above all, balance your naked lips with dramatic, smoky eyes.

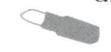

"Is there such a thing as the perfect red lipstick?"

There is a different perfect red lipstick for everyone. To find yours, ignore the color on the packaging and how it looks in the tube. Instead of testing it on the back of your hand, use the pad of your fingertip, which is closer to your natural lip color.

"Is there a rule to finding a lipstick for your hair color?"

Redheads with fair skin should choose beige or apricot.

Blondes who don't tan easily should choose coral and pinky shades.

Brunettes with olive skin need a hint of red.

Those with dark skins and hair should choose anything with a hint of gold.

"How can I make my lips look fuller?"

Don't even think about drawing lip liner above the natural curve of your lips in an attempt to create the look of an enlarged cupid's bow. Instead, use a thin brush to sweep some highlighter along the upper lip after applying a matt lip tint.

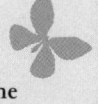
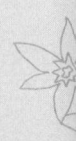

"How can I get nude lips to work in the evening?"

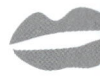

Once you've established your matt base color, rub some iridescent eye shadow over your lips to give a shimmer that is subtler than full-on gloss.

"Which lipstick colors will make my lips look bigger?"

If your pout is on the puny side, avoid dark and berry shades and go for more bold, red colors. High shine from either balm or gloss will also make them look plumper, as will dotting a bit of iridescent powder across the top of your cupid's bow.

"How can I make my big lips look smaller?"

Most women want to plump up their lips, but if you want to reduce the appearance of yours, draw the focus away from them by using a dark lipstick color.

"Will lip gloss make my lips look plumper?"

Gloss reflects the light, making lips look fuller. To maximize the effect, apply a dot of gloss in the middle of each lip, rather than all over, to create the illusion of pout-perfect lips.

"How can I get more from my make-up without breaking the bank?"

Buy a white lip gloss. It works well on its own or can transform your lipsticks into lighter, pastel-like shades when you feel like a change.

"Lipstick: one coat or two?"

Two (and a bit). Apply your first coat, blot on a tissue then dust loose powder over your lips before applying the second coat.

"When is it time to buy a new shade of lipstick?"

Be aware of the changes to your face as you age. A lighter lip shade may be more flattering to thinner lips, and using a lipstick with a blue undertone will make your teeth look whiter if they've become stained.

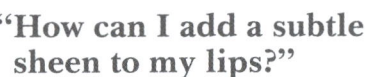

"How can I add a subtle sheen to my lips?"

Mix some liquid highlighter with some plain lip balm and smooth over your lips.

"How can I avoid making red lips look brash?"

Dilute the effect by applying a layer of clear lip balm and blending your lipstick over the top with your fingers.

APPLYING MAKE-UP 161

"Is there any way to get my hands on my favorite lipstick if the manufacturer has discontinued it?"

If you're really desperate, www.threecustom.com is a New York-based company that keeps a bank of discontinued colors of all kinds of cosmetics. Failing that, you can send them a sample and they'll remake your lipstick for you, and keep it on file for when you need some more.

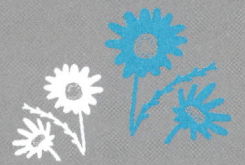

Treat yourself

"Will extensions damage my nails?"

Some salons use a cheap adhesive called monomer methyl methacrylate (MMA) to glue the acrylic extensions in place. Because it doesn't stick to the natural nail surface effectively, technicians often resort to using an electric file to shred the nail's surface, making it thinner and weaker. Be alert for a strong, unpleasant-smelling glue, a tell-tale sign of MMA.

"How can I make the curl in my lashes last longer?"

Hair perming may have gone out in the 80s, but using the same technique on your lashes is very much in. A salon therapist will apply perming solution (it smells like rotten eggs) to curl your lashes around mini curlers and leave them to set for about half an hour. The curl can last for up to six weeks.

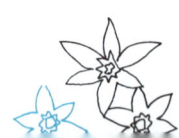

"When's the best time to have a spray tan?"

Last thing at night (preferably when it's dark outside). Wear your oldest, grubbiest tracksuit and some dark sunglasses for when you come out. The tan may come off on your clothes and your face might look like an orangutan immediately after. Don't shower until the next morning.

"Is there a pain-free treatment for cellulite?"

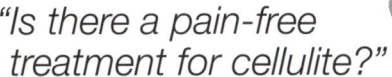

The top dermatologists are now using carbon dioxide. Carboxytherapy uses CO_2 to blast fat cells and increase blood flow to the problem area and eliminate excess fluid retention. It'll take 15 to 20 sessions of about 15 minutes, but you can start to see the effects after the first five.

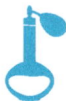

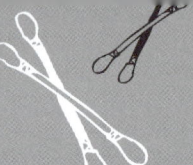

"How can I shift the cellulite on my thighs?"

Lipomassage® is a treatment involving motorized rollers to target specific orange peel areas and pummel the skin vigorously. Using movements that roll in (for areas of dense fat), out (on loose areas of skin), and upward (to recontour the legs), it claims to burn the fat and give you smoother thighs. Each session lasts 35 minutes and you'll need at least six.

"How can I blast my cellulite in time for the bikini season?"

The French technique endermologie was originally a deep-tissue massage for horses, but is now used as a temporary cellulite-busting treatment on humans. It involves using a massage machine to roll and suction the skin, break down the subcutaneous fat and release toxins. The full treatment comprises 14 sessions.

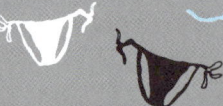

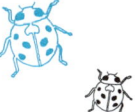

"Is there a high-tech way to tackle cellulite without surgery?"

Velasmooth® is a noninvasive, nonsurgical method that uses elios technology to beat the orange peel effect. A combination of radio frequency, optical energy and infrared light is used to increase oxygen to the skin's cells as they are massaged by rollers to smooth out the skin.

"How can I get a peachy-smooth bottom?"

Treat yourself to a butt facial. Just like an ordinary facial, it includes cleansing the skin of impurities, exfoliating dead skin cells, and an intensive moisture mask. Added into the facial is some kind of cellulite treatment to improve skin tone.

"Is there a treatment to aid weight loss?"

Food cravings are a killer for most dieters. Hypnopuncture involves having small metal seeds inserted into your ear to stimulate specific pressure points. These points promote the release of certain brain chemicals, as if you have just eaten a meal. After the treatment, you can press on these seeds to create the same effect and eliminate your cravings.

"How can I get instant weight loss?"

When there's no time for diets and it's too late for crunches, a universal wrap will have you swaddled up in muslin strips like a mummy. The muslin is applied to flatten and lift your saggy parts while elements such as clay draw out toxins from the skin and eliminate excess weight caused by water retention.

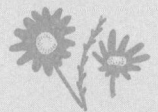

"What's the easiest way to beat cravings and stick to my diet?"

Hypnosis is an alternative method of assisting weight loss. Your therapist may be able to determine the emotional or psychological problems causing your overeating and work on your mind so that you no longer use food as a way of dealing with them.

"Which treatments are based around natural products?"

Apitherapy uses the natural healing and antibacterial properties of bee products (such as honey, beeswax, royal jelly, and bee venom) to remedy everything from allergies and cardiovascular disorders to back and neck pain.

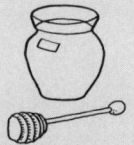

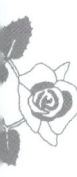

"What is phytotherapy?"

This involves the use of herbs in various forms, such as teas, oils, and ointments, which have a healing effect on the body.

"What kind of treatments can I expect to find on vacation in Indonesia?"

If you're traveling to Indonesia, Lulur is a treatment that has been used by the natives since ancient times. It combines aromatherapy massage with yogurt and flower applications and herb baths to cleanse and moisturize the skin. It is a deeply relaxing treatment if you want to pamper yourself.

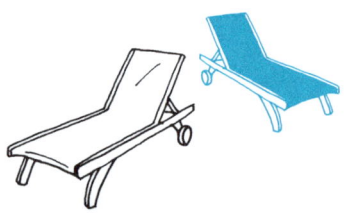

"What's a good treatment when the skin on the body is dry?"

A salt glow is one of the most popular treatments. Your therapist will apply a mixture of sea salt (to exfoliate away the dead skin cells) and moisturizing oils such as lemon, almond, or lavender, to revive your scaly skin.

"What's a body wrap?"

A treatment where you get wrapped up like a mummy, but detox and reduce fluid retention for your trouble. There are different types of wrap, but you'll generally be smothered in a thick clay, seaweed, mud, or algae, bundled up in blankets, foils, or towels and left for about 20 minutes to encourage the skin to release toxins.

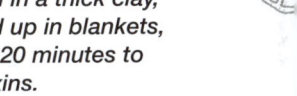

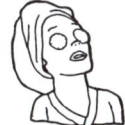

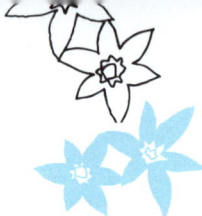

"How do I know what type of spa is right for me?"

Of all the many types of spas a beauty spa will focus on pampering and grooming treatments; a medispa will combine orthodox and alternative medicine to treat your overall health and well-being; and a cosmedispa will specialize in cosmetic surgery procedures. Resort, health, and hotel spas (as opposed to day spas) may tailor nutrition and exercise plans to the guest throughout their stay, and the new bootcamp or detox spas will ensure that there are no slackers when it comes to losing weight.

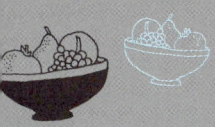

"Is spa food all wheatgrass shots and starvation?"

Not at all. Most spas serve healthy, nutritionally balanced meals that are not only delicious but also low in sugar and fat. Many spas offer the opportunity of a detox where you confine yourself to fruit and vegetable juices for a few days as a means of cleansing your system.

"Do I need to take anything when visiting a spa?"

Most spas provide everything you need (towels, robes, slippers, and water). However, if you're going to a salon for a pedicure, remember to take your flip-flops to wear afterward so you don't smudge your beautiful toes.

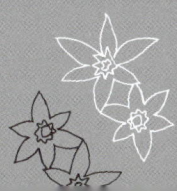

"Are all spa treatments done in therapy rooms?"

No. If you want somewhere more inspiring than your average treatment room, anthotherapy is a massage in a cave, for example. The caves are heated by hot springs or volcanic rocks nearby, creating a humid environment that assists the release of muscular tension.

"What unusual ingredients are used in spa treatments?"

Natural peat is used in body masks and baths for its ability to detoxify the skin, heal scars and blemishes, and soothe eczema.

"How can I put the oomph back into my bust?"

Why not try a bust wrap, designed to tackle the sag and crêpe with serums, lotions, and masks to firm and tone the skin. They're great for mature skins or if you've just finished breastfeeding.

"Can I take my teenage daughter to a spa?"

Many spas now offer treatments tailored to young girls, including mini manicures and facials. Visit www.spafinder.com to search for children-friendly spas and treatments for teens.

"Which treatments should I avoid during pregnancy?"

Saunas and steam rooms are generally out, as are wraps and anything that involves lying on your back for too long. Some women avoid treatments altogether in the first trimester.

"Which spa treatments can I have during pregnancy?"

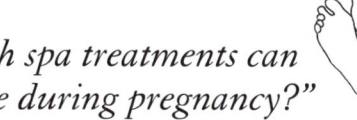

Foot treatments, including pedicures and reflexology, are a good option for tired feet and swollen ankles to sooth your ankles and help you relax. Always seek medical advice first in pregnancy.

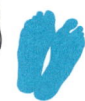

"What's an indigenous spa treatment?"

When local oils, herbs, or other plants from places such as Thailand, Hawaii, or the Caribbean are used and incorporated into the treatment.

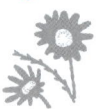

"What treatment should I choose for very dry, flaky skin?"

Try a dulse scrub, a vigorous scrub using dulse (seaweed) to scour off those scales and nourish the skin with vital vitamins and minerals.

"Are there any treatments that help with arthritis?"

A Parafango combines volcanic mud with paraffin to create a warm pack to ease the associated aches and pains.

"What's baineotherapy?"

The term for a variety of treatments that use good old H_2O (usually springwater containing minerals and salts) to draw toxins from the body, soothe the skin, and ease aches and pains.

"Is chocolate bad for my skin?"

On the contrary: good-quality chocolate is now used in some spa treatments. Cocoa butter is rich in fatty acids to soften the skin and contains glycerides, which deliver moisturizing lipids to make skin plump and firm.

"How can I treat myself and look after the environment?"

Carbon-neutral pampering is now all the rage. The latest spas offer eco-friendly pampering vacations by doing everything from relying on solar panels for energy to recycling their waste and basing their menu entirely around local and seasonal ingredients.

"What's the difference between a steam room and a sauna?"

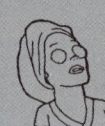

The heat in a sauna is dry, while the heat in a steam room is more humid as it comes from heating water until it evaporates.

"Why are saunas good for you?"

A sauna encourages the veins near the skin's surface to dilate, increasing circulation here and encouraging your body to sweat. This can be a good way of detoxing but it may not be suitable for pregnant women or those with high blood pressure or a heart condition. Always seek advice.

"I can't stand the heat in saunas. Is there any other way of getting the benefits?"

If you can't stand the heat, get out of the sauna. Instead, look out for a tropicarium, a cross between a sauna and a steam room where the heat is less intense.

"Are there any alternatives to a steam room?"

A Rasul bath is like a steam room crossed with a cleansing treatment. It allows you to slather yourself in different types of mud, which is absorbed into the skin and encourages your body to sweat.

"What's Ayurveda?"

An ancient Indian practice that aims to create harmony within the body by understanding the individual energy types of dosha. Your dosha (either vata, pitta, or kapha) determines the type of lifestyle you lead, the foods you should eat, the exercise that suits you best, any homeopathic supplements you could take, and helpful treatments.

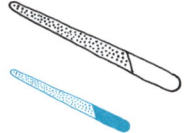

"How can I find a good treatment to relax me?"

Follow Ayurvedic principles, which seek to balance physical and mental health, and opt for a Shirodhara. The name comes from two words meaning *head* and *flow* and the treatment involves having warm oil poured onto the middle of your forehead, followed by a scalp (and sometimes body) massage. Many people find it so relaxing they fall asleep during the treatment and maintain a feeling of inner calm for days afterward.

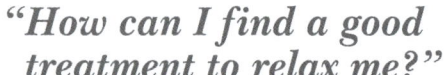

"Are there any treatments to help me sleep?"

For water babies, flotation is perfect. Lie inside a pod of shallow water containing mineral salts that support your body weight, causing a feeling of dreamlike weightlessness. It's ideal for people who don't like the intimacy of a massage or have muscular and joint strains. The minerals are also good for your skin and it'll help you get a good night's sleep.

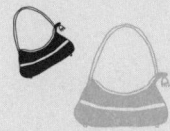

"What on earth is fangotherapy?"

It comes from the Italian word *fango*, meaning mud. During the treatment, a clay-based mud with added ingredients such as marine algae, herbs, or essential oils is applied to the body to absorb excess sebum, draw out toxins, soften the skin, and relieve aches and pains.

"Are there treatments to cure migraines?"

Craniosacral therapy has been successfully used in the treatment of migraines and can also help with pain and stress relief. The practitioner works to bring about subtle shifts in the spinal and cranial bones to rebalance the central nervous system and ease restrictions in the nerve passages.

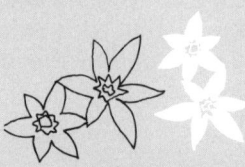

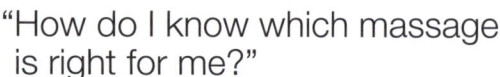

"How do I know which massage is right for me?"

Massages work on the lymphatic, muscular, and nervous systems, but different types will serve different needs. Lymphatic drainage massage is a deep-tissue massage where pressure from the thumb is applied in sweeping strokes to increase lymphatic flow, essential in supporting the immune system. It improves circulation, boosts immunity, helps with cellulite and toxin elimination, and reduces fluid retention. A Thai massage fuses Eastern techniques, from yoga to acupressure and reflexology and is good for rebalancing the mind and body. A Swedish massage combines pressure and stretching in five basic strokes. It's good for releasing toxins and easing post-exercise muscular soreness.

"What's an aromatherapy massage?"

An aromatherapy massage uses aromatherapy oils to ease muscle tension, nourish the skin, and uplift or calm the mind. Good for relaxation and reenergizing.

"Are massages safe during pregnancy?"

Many spas now offer specially tailored prenatal massages that may have you lying on cushions or beanbags, rather than traditional therapy beds, to support you and your bump in a comfortable position. It's best to book a special pregnancy massage rather than go for a regular one.

"Will a massage hurt?"

While most will not, deep tissue and sports massages involve a thorough (and often painful) kneading of the muscles to relieve tension. Not for anyone who wants relaxation.

"What on earth is a pizzichilli?"

It may sound like something you'd order in an Italian restaurant, but it's actually a deeply relaxing treatment in which two therapists pour warm oil all over your body and massage it into your skin.

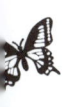

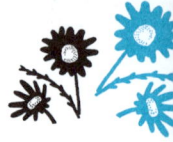

"What's a Shiatsu massage?"

Traditional Chinese medicine works on the belief that, over time, our natural energy paths become blocked, causing emotional and physical imbalance. Shiatsu is a bit like acupuncture without the needles and works to free these blockages by combining massage on key pressure points with stretching. It's good for stimulating the immune system, detoxification, aiding restful sleep, and easing sore muscles and joints.

"What's a great all-round massage?"

A Mandara treatment can blend several different styles of massage (including Japanese, Shiatsu, Thai, Swedish, Lomi Lomi, and Balinese), with two or three therapists working on you simultaneously.

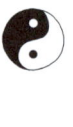
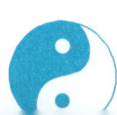

"Which treatments will reenergize me?"

During a crystal massage, the therapist places quartz crystals at strategic points along your back. It's an ancient method of releasing tension and energy blockages and promoting self-healing.

"Are there any treatments that are good for damaged or broken skin?"

A Traeger massage (named after its inventor, Dr. Milton Traeger) uses no oils or rubbing and you keep your clothes on throughout. Instead, it involves gentle rocking movements that nurture the body and help relieve tension and joint pain.

"What's rolfing?"

A treatment not for the faint-hearted, which uses deep massage to improve musculoskeletal alignment, including your posture.

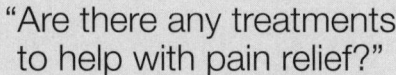

"Are there any treatments to help with pain relief?"

In the Bowen Technique, the therapist massages the skin beneath thumb and forefinger in a rolling motion to prompt the body to rebalance and heal itself. It can be helpful for everything from back and neck pain to sports injuries and chronic fatigue.

"How does reflexology work?"

Reflexology dates back to Ancient India, Egypt, and China and works on the basis that certain points on the feet correspond to different organs in the body. By stimulating these points, the practitioner can help ease symptoms associated with everything from digestive problems to stress, migraines, pain, infertility, and hormonal imbalances.

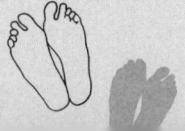

"Are there any treatments that help clear a cold?"

Take a visit to a eucalyptus oil aroma room. It's a bit like a having a scented sauna to clear the sinuses.

"What's a good treatment for aches and pains?"

Don some plastic underpants and sink into a paraffin bath. The warm paraffin helps relieve aches, softens your skin, and reduces water retention in the body.

"Is there a good treatment for scaly, winter skin?"

Brossage is a body polishing treatment using lots of small, soft-bristled brushes and salicylic salt to exfoliate and brighten the skin.

"What is a Panthermal treatment?"

Panthermal requires you to lie in a metal tube with your head poking out. The tube is piped full of hot, dry air, which engulfs the body and makes you sweat. This is followed by soapy jets of water that pummel you from all directions to help break down cellulite.

"What's cupping?"

Remember Gwyneth Paltrow's red-ringed back when she attended a celeb party a few years ago? That was the aftermath of cupping, a technique from traditional Chinese medicine that involves placing heated glass jars on the skin to create a vacuum. It flushes excess fluid and toxins from the muscles, stimulates the nervous system and blood flow to the skin and induces a feeling of overall well-being.

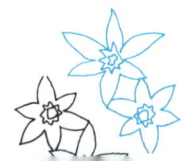

"What's reiki?"

This gentle massage originated in Tibet more than 2,500 years ago and can has been found to alleviate stress and even promote healing for people suffering chronic physical illnesses. The treatment aims to restore physical, mental, and spiritual balance by allowing our individual qi, or energy, to flow freely through us.

"What should I look for in a facial?"

Different types of facial will cover everything from extraction (squeezing pores and blackheads) to exfoliation, deep cleansing, moisturizing, and toning. If you can't afford a really expensive one, choose a simple facial that includes a long massage with essential oils to increase circulation and give your skin an instant boost.

"What's the best preparty facial?"

Avoid anything with extraction (squeezing the dirt out of your pores, sure to leave you red and blotchy) and go for a lymphatic drainage treatment to reduce puffiness and act like an instant (if short-term) face-lift.

"How often should I have a facial?"

No facial is ever going to have permanent results. The frequency of your treatments will depend on your skin type (very dry and oily types might need more frequent attention) and whether you live in a city, where there is more pollution. Generally, one every six weeks should keep skin in good condition.

"Will my facial be relaxing?"

It depends on the type of facial you go for: some include painful squeezing and extraction, others don't.

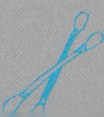

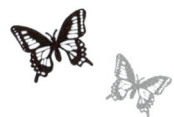

"Why does Madonna love oxygen facials?"

Madonna is just one of many celebs who are addicted to oxygen facials. The theory is that due to the aging process and environmental factors, skin can become deprived of sufficient oxygen. An oxygen facial uses a special gadget to replenish the skin's O_2 levels, making it look temporarily healthier and plumper.

"How can I get an instant lift before a night on the town?"

Try a cryogenic facial. A cocktail of vitamins and other skin-boosters is applied using a special wand that has been cooled below freezing. An increased amount of oxygen is supplied to the skin, allowing it to absorb the vitamins and appear instantly plumper.

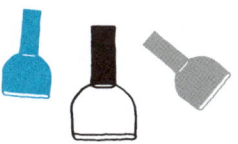

"What's a good way to deal with milia?"

Milia are raised, off-white spots around the eyes or cheekbones. Normally, the skin exfoliates itself but moisturizers, make-up, and other products can cause dead cells to become trapped under the surface, forming the white beads. Combating milia is best done by a salon professional who will pierce the bead with a sterilized needle then apply gentle pressure to unblock the pore.

"Will microdermabrasion make my skin look younger?"

This treatment is like sandblasting for the skin, usually with crystals or a diamond-tipped wand. It removes the upper layer of dead skin cells, vacuum cleans the pores and stimulates new collagen growth, and produces a noticeable difference immediately. It's perfect for people with sun-damaged skin, acne scarring, and the early signs of fine lines. If your wrinkles are already deeply etched, it's unlikely to make a dramatic difference.

"How long does a course of microdermabrasion take?"

It takes about three months of sessions every two to three weeks to see results, so start early. Make the last appointment a few days before the party to make sure you have no traces of redness.

"When's the best time to have a face peel?"

Salon peels, which use a fairly high concentration of acid, require you to stay out of the sun for a few days. It's best to have these done in fall or winter and use lower-strength home peels in the spring and summer.

"Are all chemical peels the same?"

There are several different types, which vary in the depth of the skin they penetrate. Lactic and glycolic acid peels are more superficial, while beta hydroxy and Jessner's peels act more deeply beneath the skin's surface.

"Is there a totally noninvasive treatment to erase facial wrinkles?"

Thermage is knife- and needle-free. It works by heating the web of collagen beneath the upper layer of the skin, causing collagen renewal and immediate tightening of the skin. There's no recovery time and the results may even develop in the six months after having the treatment.

"How can I make the lines on my forehead less obvious?"

Consider getting a new haircut. A chin-length bob and bangs can do wonders when it comes to framing and slimming your face and concealing lines.

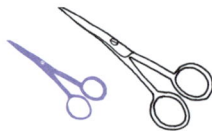

"How can I make my eyes look younger?"

It's not only the hair on our heads that thins as we age, our eyelashes do too. For bright, wide-awake eyes, treat yourself to some eyelash extensions, which bond individual synthetic lashes to your own and can for last up to two months.

"How can I tone up my face without going under the knife?"

Myotonology does just that by delivering microcurrents to isolated muscles to cause minute contractions and increase circulation to the skin. You are able to see results 24 to 48 hours after the treatment, but a course of treatments has a cumulative effect that lasts longer.

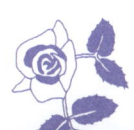

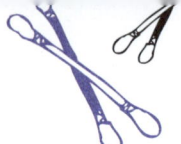

"Can I get a face-lift without surgery?"

The CACI (computer-aided cosmetology instrument) facial calls itself the "nonsurgical face-lift" and uses electrical impulses to stimulate muscle tone in the skin. It claims to lessen the appearance of wrinkles, reduce large pores, and help blemished skin.

"What's the best method for permanent hair removal?"

Permanent in this instance does not actually mean permanent, but long-term methods will last for about a year. Electrolysis involves a thin metal wand being inserted into the hair follicle. It delivers electricity to the follicle and damages it to stop it from producing more hair. It is successful, but it does hurt (a lot) and you may still get regrowth after a while.

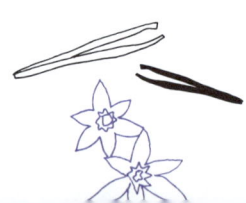

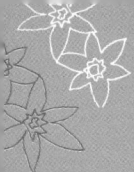

"Is laser hair removal worth it?"

This involves light of a specific wavelength being used to damage the hair follicle but leave the surrounding tissue unharmed. You're likely to get regrowth after a while, but it should be finer and lighter. This is good for people with bothersome dark hair.

"How can I make my salon waxes more bearable?"

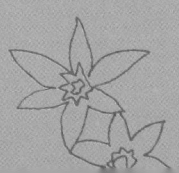

Look for Lycon® waxing, a type of hot wax that comes in blends of lavender and camomile or chocolate and hazelnut to make it feel more soothing and luxurious. The wax shrinkwraps the hair but avoids the skin, minimizing your chances of in-grown hairs, bruising, redness, or sensitivity.

"Why do I get sensitivity after waxing?"

Not only could the wax be causing the reaction on your skin, but if you're using products containing retinol, your skin will be ultrasensitive. Cut out the retinol a week before and after waxing and avoid sun exposure near the time of your appointment.

"What's the best way to remove hair when my skin is sensitive?"

Try sugaring, a technique that originated in Egypt. The mixture of sugar, lemon juice, and water adheres only to the hair, rather than the skin as waxing does. The hair is pulled out from the root but the syrup contains no harsh chemicals and is kinder to sensitive skin.

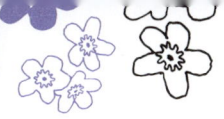

"Is there a painless method of permanent hair removal?"

Erayser® Hair Removal works by using intense pulsed light of various wavelengths and a light-sensitive lotion to destroy the hair root. It can be used to treat any skin type without side effects and it's painless, so there's no need for cooling gels. Hair regrowth can stop altogether after six treatments.

"How can I maximize the time between salon waxing appointments?"

Epilar®, a treatment available in salons, involves massaging an inhibitor and activator gel into the skin for one minute each after your normal wax. It can double regrowth time and reduce the number of hairs by up to 20 percent.

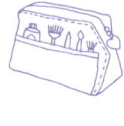
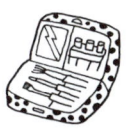

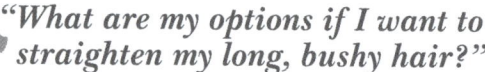

"What are my options if I want to straighten my long, bushy hair?"

Using straighteners every day will leave it dry and damaged, and although a professional blow-dry will leave it sleek and shiny for days, this can be expensive when done on a weekly basis. Your best option is the latest permanent straightening treatment from Japan. Thermal reconditioning restructures the hair's protein bonds from the inside out, leaving it absolutely straight for up to six months.

"How can I skip blow-drying but still get a great hairstyle?"

Air styling is the latest salon way to style hair without the damaging effects of heat. After washing, a stylist whips his fingers through your hair in a series of speedy strokes, removing the moisture and dampness from the hair. It's most effective on short to mid-length hair with layers and can create extra volume to flat hair.

"What if I hate my new hair color?"

Hair stripping, or color correction, is an intense method that uses bleach to make the hair more porous, allowing the color to be removed. The result is an ashy blonde, but your colorist may add another dye to achieve the color you want to achieve. Stripping shouldn't be done regularly because it can weaken the hair.

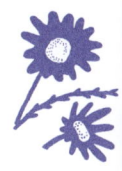

"What kind of haircut will flatter a fuller face?"

Avoid anything too long or too short and go for a mid-length style with some soft, long layers to elongate your face.

"How can I pamper my hair?"

If facials aren't your thing, "hair spas" are now all the rage. Many salons are opening up separate areas away from the hustle and bustle of the blow-dryers, to create a peaceful, relaxing environment dedicated entirely to hair treatments and scalp massages.

"How can I keep my brittle, colored hair healthy?"

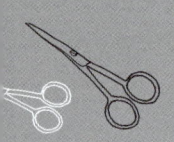

Intersperse keratin *shots* between your color appointments. It'll repair your damaged hair and boost its shine.

"How can I use my hairstyle to conceal my stick-out ears?"

Avoid short, sleek bobs (your ears will only poke out) and opt for a midlength with volume-boosting layers at the sides.

"Should I buy specialist hair products from my salon?"

They may be pricey but salon products are often the most effective, particularly if you color your hair. Red fades fastest, so buy a conditioning color booster from the salon to keep you going until your next appointment.

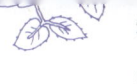

"How can I give my fine hair more shape?"

A shorter cut will instantly give your hair a boost. Dry it with a round brush, pulling outward rather than downward for more volume.

"How long before a big event should I book a hair appointment?"

Book a cut and color a week in advance to give it time to settle in. If you're feeling extravagant, have a treatment and blow-dry on the day itself. If you're having your hair put up, never arrive with newly washed hair because it is more difficult to style.

"What are the different types of hair extensions?"

Clip-ons are attached to your hair temporarily, bonding/sealing extensions are braided and bonded into your natural hair, while fusions are fused to your own hair using warm protein.

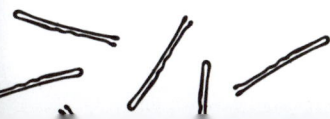

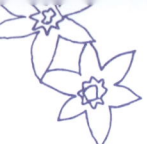

"Which type of hair extension is best for very fine hair?"

Cold fusion uses a gentle protein-based polymer to attach the extensions to your roots. The lack of heat means it's kinder to fine hair.

"Will extensions damage my hair?"

Not if they are done by an experienced professional and you follow their aftercare advice.

"Can I treat my hair as normal after having hair extensions?"

You can wash it as normal (although avoid silicone- and sulfur-based products), go swimming, and use styling tools. Just don't use a hot hairdryer, strengtheners, or curling irons near the bonds because they'll melt!

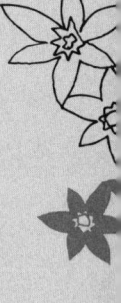

"Is there a treatment to combat bad breath?"

Tooth whitening has been all the rage for years now, but for those who want to beat bad breath at the same time, the latest technology from California allows dentists to analyze the cause of your problem and tailor a treatment to deal with it. They can polish your teeth at the same time so your pearly whites match your new fresh breath.

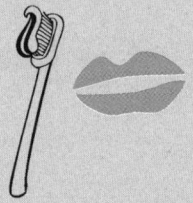
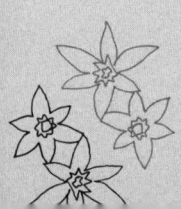

Surgical intervention

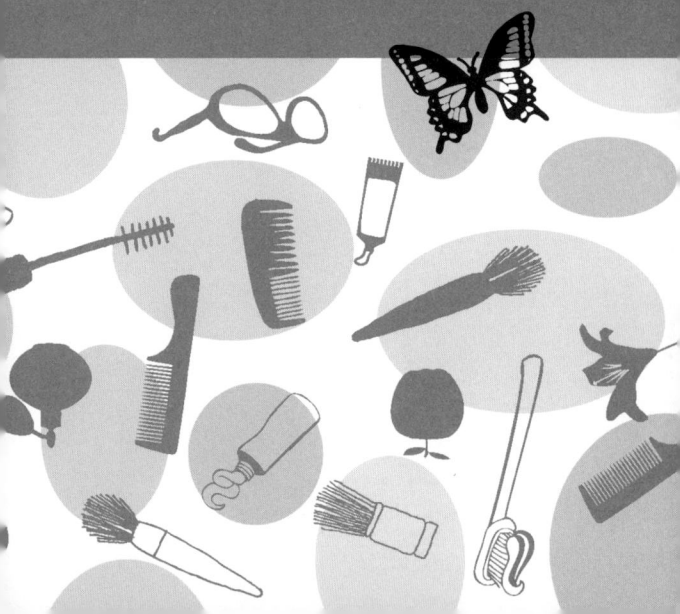

"How can you tell if someone has had cosmetic surgery?"

The dead-giveaways are as follows:

Mobile hairline: during a face- or brow-lift, the skin is pulled upward, pushing the hairline back.

Tell-tale scars: usually behind the ears after face-lifts and on the chin after facial liposuction.

Ridged lips: trout pouts are the extreme but a thin line of filler along the ridge of the lips also gives the game away.

Botox brow: when the tips jut menacingly upward.

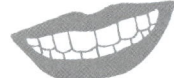

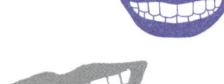

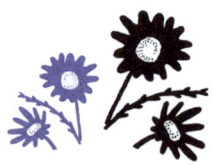

"How can I minimize scarring after surgery?"

Plastic surgeons in the United Kingdom have come up with a new miracle product called Heal, which does exactly what its name suggests. Used after surgery, it can reduce inflammation, help the skin to repair itself and reduce recovery time overall.

"Is cosmetic surgery cheaper abroad?"

The medical tourism industry (when patients seek plastic surgery in other countries) is booming. You can often save money, but always ensure you have a reputable surgeon and have medical travel insurance to cover both the medical and travel elements of your trip.

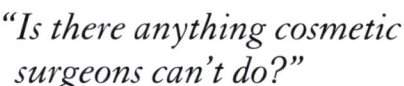

"Is there anything cosmetic surgeons can't do?"

Surgery techniques are getting more and more advanced. One of the latest procedures is the 'designer vagina' (or Designer Laser Vaginoplasty®), which improves the shape, size, and proportion of the vulva.

"I haven't got the time or skill for a proper make-up routine. Can you suggest some short cuts?"

Permanent make-up, or micropigmentation, is a cosmetic process that can do everything from coloring your brows to adding definition to your lips. If this sounds too scary, most salons offer eyelash tinting and perming using dyes and miniature hair curlers. You'll wake up each morning looking like a bright-eyed china doll.

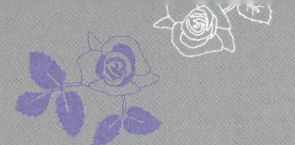

"How does permanent make-up work?"

In micropigmentation, pigment is embedded in the skin to add color, defining the lips, eyes or brows, or creating a permanent effect of blusher or eye shadow. There is also semi-permanent make-up, which lasts three to five years.

"Is permanent make-up safe?"

You are effectively tattooing your face and there have been incidences of inflammation, swelling, cracking, peeling, blistering, and infection, especially around the eye. No cosmetic surgery procedures are without risk.

"Is there a face-lift available with little or no downtime?"

While a traditional face-lift will leave you hospital-bound for a night and home-bound for many more, contour threading takes only 40 to 90 minutes and enables you to return to work in a day or two. During the procedure, tiny threads are inserted beneath the hairline to lift sagging skin and rebalance facial symmetry.

"Will a face-lift leave me with scars?"

Traditional face-lifts leave a scar behind the ears, making some hairstyles a no-no. Surgeons are now working on scarless face-lifts, which leave only invisible scars beneath the hairline and inside the mouth.

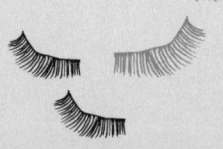

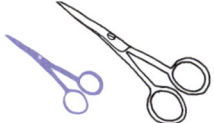

"What's the latest in face-lifts?"

Not content with rearranging the skin to make us look younger, surgeons are now looking to realign the bones of the skull that support the skin from underneath.

"Is there an alternative to chemical peels?"

Like a chemical peel, laser resurfacing removes the upper layers of skin to reveal smoother, wrinkle-free ones beneath. Instead of chemicals, it uses carbon dioxide to vaporize these layers and is done under a local anesthetic and sedation.

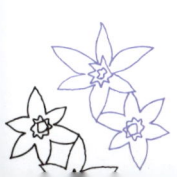

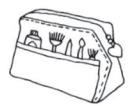

"What can I do about the spidery red broken capillaries on my cheeks?"

A course of four to eight intense pulse light (IPL) treatments will work through a process called photo rejuvenation. Pulses of light are beamed onto the skin after a cold gel has been applied. The light works on the excess hemoglobin, destroying the redness.

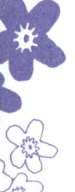

"Is there any kind of treatment that can make acne vanish?"

If you've got a hot date or really just can't wait to get rid of that enormous pimple, a cortisone injection administered by a dermatologist will banish it fast by reducing the swelling and redness.

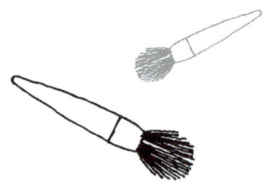

"Are there any surgical procedures for acne?"

For severe cases of acne that don't respond to topical creams or medicine, Isolaz deep pore laser therapy is a new treatment that combines a vacuum action with laser to destroy the bacteria that cause the acne. You can see results after four sessions of ten minutes.

"What's the procedure for removing eye bags?"

Blepharoplasty involves making an incision in the natural crease of the upper and/or lower eyelid to remove excess fat and sagging muscle and skin. The under-eye areas can then be gently lifted before closing the incisions. Surgery can take up to three hours and it may be ten days before most of the bruising and swelling has subsided.

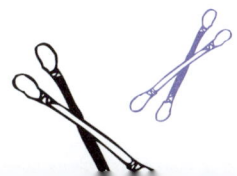

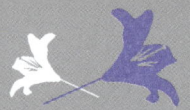

"How can I get bigger brows?"

Eyebrow transplants are now available for those who are a little sparse up top. The procedure takes three to four hours and is done to match your natural hair color, giving a more realistic effect than tattooing and permanent make-up techniques.

"Are all wrinkles the same?"

They may look similar, but actually there are different types. Expression lines (crow's feet and lines between the brows) are caused by muscle contractions that move the skin. Fine lines (such as those under the eye) occur due to gradual loss of elasticity as the skin ages. Static lines are unrelated to muscle movement.

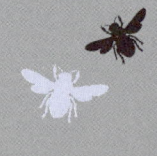

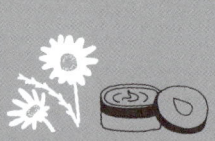

"Other than needles or the knife, what are the options for erasing wrinkles?"

Omnilux is a light therapy that uses specific wavelengths to stimulate collagen production. It's not painful, requires no recovery time, and will usually last 30 to 45 minutes for each session.

"What's the best antiwrinkle procedure when I need results fast?"

Restylane SubQ® is a Swedish filler that celebs rely on to keep their faces shapely, particularly before a big event. It is made from hyarulonic acid and recontours the face rather than just filling lines. You'll need a local anesthetic, but the whole thing will be done before your lunch hour is over.

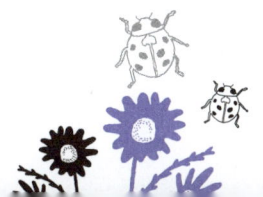

"Can I fix my wrinkles in one shot?"

Evolence® is a new filler that, unlike Botox®, may smooth out your lines in just one jab. It's made from natural collagen to support the skin's structure, making it look plumper and stronger.

"What does the future hold for antiaging procedures?"

The sky's the limit, but some dermatologists and endocrinologists are working on using human growth hormone as a way to ward off wrinkles, increase energy levels, and boost metabolic rate. It's highly controversial and not licenced for use in this way, but some doctors are prescribing it privately. Misuse of the hormone or contaminated versions can lead to bloating, swelling, excessive growth, and even adrenal failure.

SURGICAL INTERVENTION 219

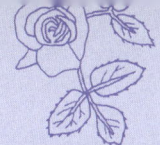

"What is collagen?"

It's a protein produced in the body that acts as its main connective tissue. Over time, the amount of collagen in the body decreases, causing visible signs of aging like wrinkles.

"How do dermal fillers differ from collagen treatments?"

Dermal fillers, such as Restylane® and Hydrafill®, add volume to sagging skin by attracting water and hydrating it. Collagen treatments restore the skin's structure by restocking the collagen that has been lost over time.

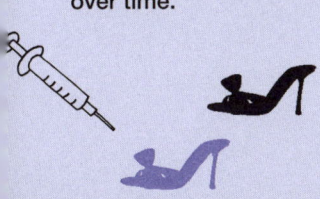

"How bad will the bruising be after a dermal filler?"

It can take up to a week for the bruising and swelling to go down. However, there is such a thing as a *magic needle* that enters the skin without damaging the dermis or breaking blood vessels, so there's no purple aftereffects.

"How can I get natural but fuller-looking lips?"

If you want plumper lips but not a trout pout, try Laresse®, a nonpermanent dermal filler that has nonanimal and nonbacterial components so is safer to use and makes for a smoother, more natural look.

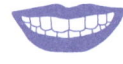
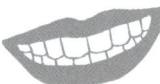
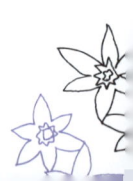

"Is there an alternative to dermal fillers?"

If you like the sound of having a smoother face, but are put off by the cocktail of ingredients that some fillers contain, try MesoGlow. A mixture of antioxidants, vitamins, minerals and amino acids are injected into the dermis through a series of needle pricks to nourish the skin and promote the production of collagen. It's recommended that you have six treatments two weeks apart, then a booster once a year.

"What's the latest filler for the lower half of the face?"

While Botox® is generally used on what surgeons call the "upper third" of the face (frown lines, forehead creases, and crow's feet), Juvederm® Ultra is used to tackle lines on the cheeks, chin, and around the mouth. Some say it's safer than Botox® because it contains hyaluronic acid, a chemical that occurs naturally in the body but depletes as we age.

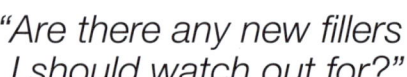

"Are there any new fillers I should watch out for?"

Launching in 2008, Reloxin® (otherwise known as Dysport) may knock Botox® from the top filler spot. It's a form of botulinum type A but is said to disperse more effectively, helping to smooth a wider area around the point where it is injected.

"What's the alternative to lip fillers?"

PermaLip® is like a boob job for the lips. Non-rupture silicon implants are inserted into the lips to make them fuller without giving the hard, unnatural look of traditional implants.

"Why do derma fillers tend to be nonpermanent?"

Our faces change in minute, nonperceivable ways every day, but over time, these changes start to become noticeable. Temporary fillers act and adapt to your face at the time of the procedure but have the advantage of breaking down before changes in the face make it look as if it's been frozen.

"Do fillers just paper over the cracks or can they be beneficial to the skin?"

NewFill (or Sculptra®) is known as a dermal-stimulating filler that not only fills in your lines but also stimulates the skin to produce collagen and subcutaneous tissue. The skin therefore starts to correct the lines itself, even when the filler breaks down.

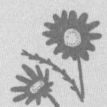

"How does Botox® work?"

Botox® (and also Dysport) are the trade names for botulinum toxin, produced by bacteria called Clostridium botulinum. *It is injected under the skin of the face and works by blocking the nerve impulses that tell the muscles to contract. It temporarily relaxes or paralyzes muscles, giving you a smoother, more youthful appearance.*

"What's the difference between having Botox® and a face-lift?"

A face-lift is an invasive procedure that involves actually cutting the skin, leaving it bruised and swollen. The swelling may take weeks to go down, but the procedure is permanent. Botox® is an injection beneath the skin at the site of the wrinkles, which freezes the muscles temporarily. You'll have minimal bruising afterward but you will need boosters every three to six months.

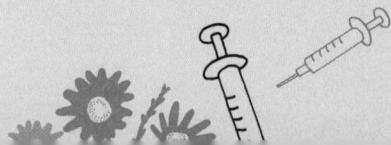

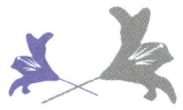

"How long after treatment before Botox® takes effect?"

About 24 to 72 hours after the injection.

"Is it safe to have Botox® during pregnancy?"

While some experts say anything injected into the face is unlikely to affect other areas of the body, others believe it's unwise to expose pregnant women to toxins in this way. In any case, pregnant women tend to hold more water, making their faces plumper and less lined, so may not need Botox® anyway.

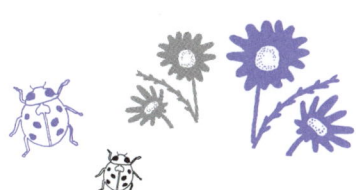

"Is there a natural alternative to Botox®?"

Artefill, or Artecoll, is a natural collagen filler that, unlike Botox®, has the advantage of not being absorbed by the body. Its effects are immediate and you'll probably need only one or two shots to work in the long term.

"Is Botox® dangerous?"

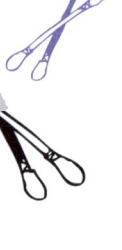

According to the FDA (Food and Drug Administration), Botox® is a lethal substance. In most cases, it is thought that the dosage is too low to cause side-effects, yet there have been reports of respiratory illnesses and even death linked to a wide range of doses. The odds are small, but it can happen, and at the very least an unskilled practitioner could leave you looking as though your face got stuck after the wind changed.

"How long will Botox® last?"

Usually three to four months.

"Is it a good idea to have a Botox® booster before a big event?"

Leave it about two weeks before your event to get the maximum results and allow any bruising to subside.

"Are there more permanent alternatives to Botox®?"

However good the initial effect of Botox®, stubborn lines can reform when it breaks down. A new procedure called SurgiWire® uses tissue from the patient's own body to fill the crease, providing much longer-lasting results.

"What other more permanent fillers are there?"

Portrait® Skin Rejuvenation is a new filler that promotes collagen growth in the deep layers of the skin, resulting in a smoother appearance on the surface. It tackles all types of wrinkles, the results improve with time, and it need only take one treatment to achieve a long-lasting difference.

"Is there a safer alternative to Botox®?"

Glabellar Furrow Relaxation is called "No-tox" by those in the know. A small probe delivers radio frequency to the muscles in the face to paralyze them, rather than using an injection. It's about ten times more expensive than Botox® and can last up to two years, which is good news if you like the outcome but bad if you don't.

"Could Botox® freeze my face permanently?"

The body breaks down Botox® after about six months, so while a botched job may cause temporary paralysis, your face will return to normal in time.

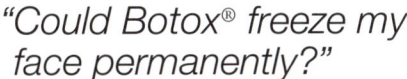

"Is there a risk of looking worse after my first treatment of Botox® wears off?"

Unlikely. Some experts even say the lines are improved because you have learnt not to use certain muscles over the period during which they have been frozen.

"Will my body *get used* to Botox®?"

People commonly fear that their bodies will become resistant to the treatment, meaning they'll need higher and higher doses each time. In fact, many surgeons actually report a softening of lines after a few treatments, so lower doses are actually required.

"Are there any other uses for Botox®?"

Yes. Excessive perspiration and migraines are other common ailments that Botox® has been used to treat.

"How will I know if I'm allergic to Botox®?"

Symptoms can range from a rash to itching, neck pain, headaches, nausea, and shortness of breath. You should seek medical advice if you experience any of these after the treatment.

"I'm allergic to Botox®. What now?"

Try Dermalogen®, a filler made from processed human skin. It is chemically identical to the collagen in your own skin and helps smooth out wrinkles but is less likely to cause an allergic reaction.

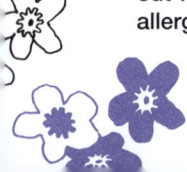

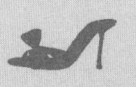

"What if I don't want to go to a clinic for my procedure?"

Look for services that come to you. Check that you are using a reputable surgeon and you could be having your wrinkles smoothed in the comfort of your own home.

"Is professional tooth whitening suitable for everyone?"

In a word, no. It's not recommended for women who are pregnant or breastfeeding, for anyone with a lot of porcelain veneers or extreme tooth discoloration. If your teeth are naturally sensitive (you get a shooting pain when you eat something hot or cold, or your teeth look slightly translucent), the agony you'll suffer will not be worth it.

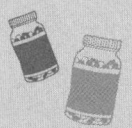

"What if professional tooth whitening makes my teeth too white?"

In Hollywood, there's no such thing as too white. However, if you don't want your teeth to glow in the dark, ask your dentist to match the color of your teeth to that of the whites of your eyes. This should produce the most natural look.

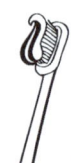

"How does professional tooth whitening differ from the dental trays you use at home?"

Most professional services work either by exposing the teeth to intense heat to activate the whitening agent gel, or by using a light-activated laser system that can lighten teeth by up to eight shades in just 45 minutes. Home treatments use hydrogen or carbamide peroxide gel and a custom-made bleaching tray, which you wear for a period of time each day (sometimes overnight). This gel contains a lower concentration of peroxide than the professional ones, so it's better for those with sensitive teeth.

"How can I get a Hollywood smile?"

Lumineers® are new porcelain veneers that are as thin as a contact lens. Unlike having traditional veneers fitted, you'll need no anesthetic. The procedure is said to be painless and noninvasive, and you'll get a perfect smile that will last up to 20 years after just two visits to the dentist.

"Is liposuction a good option for getting rid of my flabby thighs?"

Liposuction works by a practitioner inserting a narrow metal tube into the skin and sucking the fat out. Yes, your legs will be skinnier, and it is usually permanent, but it does carry the risk of infection, and you will be bruised and swollen for up to six months and have permanent scars.

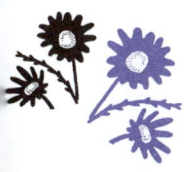

"Is there a less drastic alternative to liposuction?"

During Laser lipo, two paddles are applied to your problem area while small laser probes are placed over the lymph glands. You'll then spend ten minutes on a vibration plate to break down the fat cells, which are removed by the lymph system. Neither a local nor a general anesthetic is needed and you can lose up to 3 inches in the eight recommended sessions.

"How can I lose weight from my body but not my face?"

There was a time when women had to choose between a slim body and a gaunt face, or a fuller body and a more radiant face. Then along came F.A.M.I (Fat Auto-graft Muscle Injection), a procedure using liposuction to remove fat from the hips, then using the stem cells to plump up lines on the face.

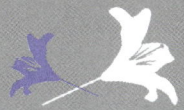

"How does a tummy tuck work?"

Otherwise known as abdominoplasty, this involves removing skin and fat from your tummy to tighten the muscles there. People who have lost a lot of weight but still have the excess skin often use this as a means of getting a flatter, smoother stomach.

"What can I do about the thread veins on my legs?"

Microscleropathy involves injecting the veins with a chemical to thicken them and make them stick together. After a week of wearing a compression stocking after the treatment, the veins will disperse naturally. They may come back after a while but you can go back for further treatment.

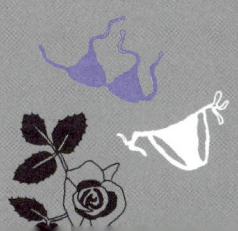

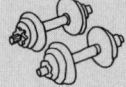
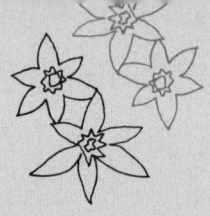

"What can I do about my sagging underarms?"

An arm lift (or brachioplasty) will reshape the underarm between your armpit and elbow, to tighten sagging skin. However, you will be left with significant scarring so it may be better to try a few tricep dips in the gym first.

"How can I get my youthful hands back?"

Being constantly exposed to the elements can leave hands looking thin and gnarled. Restylane®, a dermal filler also used to fight facial lines, can be injected into the hands to make them look plumper and smoother.

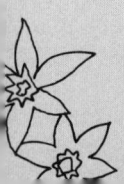
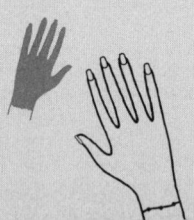

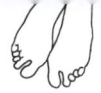

SURGICAL INTERVENTION

"How can I get dainty feet?"

There's hardly a body part untouched by cosmetic surgeons these days. Women who want feet to do their new shoes justice are now having foot lifts and toe tucks to narrow their feet and shorten their toes.

"How can I make my legs more shapely?"

Silicone calf implants are popular and can add more definition to the lower leg and balance out chunky thighs.

"How can I get a bum like J Lo's?"

Hollywood ladies have set the trend for the "butt lift," which uses fat taken from elsewhere in the body to be inserted into your behind to make it more pert and firmer.

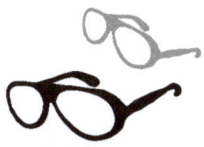

"Why are breast implants different shapes?"

The shape depends on the position of the implant and the shape of your natural breasts. Implants are usually round and come in varying widths. They may also be teardrop-shaped, making the lower half of the breast project more than the upper part. However, these may rotate over time causing asymmetry, so round ones might be a better option.

"What are the different implant options for a boob job?"

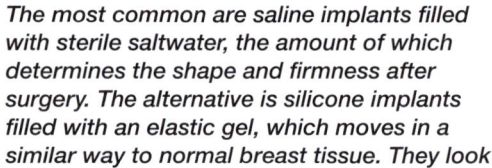

The most common are saline implants filled with sterile saltwater, the amount of which determines the shape and firmness after surgery. The alternative is silicone implants filled with an elastic gel, which moves in a similar way to normal breast tissue. They look the same, but silicone ones feel more natural.

"Do breast implants go out of date?"

While the manufacturers say they won't necessarily last a lifetime, they don't state how long they will last. Those with silicone implants are advised to have an MRI scan every two years to detect signs of rupturing, in which case you will have to have them replaced or removed.

"What happens during a boob job?"

After you are placed under general anesthetic, the surgeon makes a small incision, usually underneath the breast or armpit, or near the nipple. The implant is placed behind the pectoral muscle or behind the breast tissue. Your surgeon will help you decide beforehand which is the best option for you, depending on your anatomy and desired outcome.

"How long is the recovery period after breast augmentation?"

Usually about six weeks.

"I want to have breast implants. What's the best way to find a surgeon?"

With ladies now having lipo in their lunch hour and Botox® between meetings, unqualified practitioners are taking more risks with our health. Seek advice from an independent consultant who will shop around for a reputable practitioner to best suit your individual needs and budget.

"How can I boost my energy?"

If you feel yourself flagging, some medispas now offer vitamin B_{12} injections, which promise to revive your energy levels after six days or so.

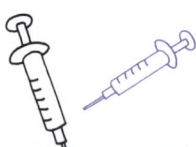

"Are there any other breast augmentation alternatives to a boob job?"

Macrolane® is the new wonder invention that claims to be a boob job in a jab. There's no general anesthetic or surgery and it leaves only small scars. A tiny incision is made beneath each breast so that a gel filler of hyaluronic acid (a substance that occurs naturally in the body) can be pumped into it. It creates a more subtle boost but the filler does break down after a year, so you'll need refills.

"What's the latest way to get rid of a tattoo?"

Scientists are working on a carbon dioxide-based laser that targets the deep layers of skin to erase tattoos but causes minimal damage to the skin. Unlike some traditional laser procedures, it can also be done on an outpatient basis.

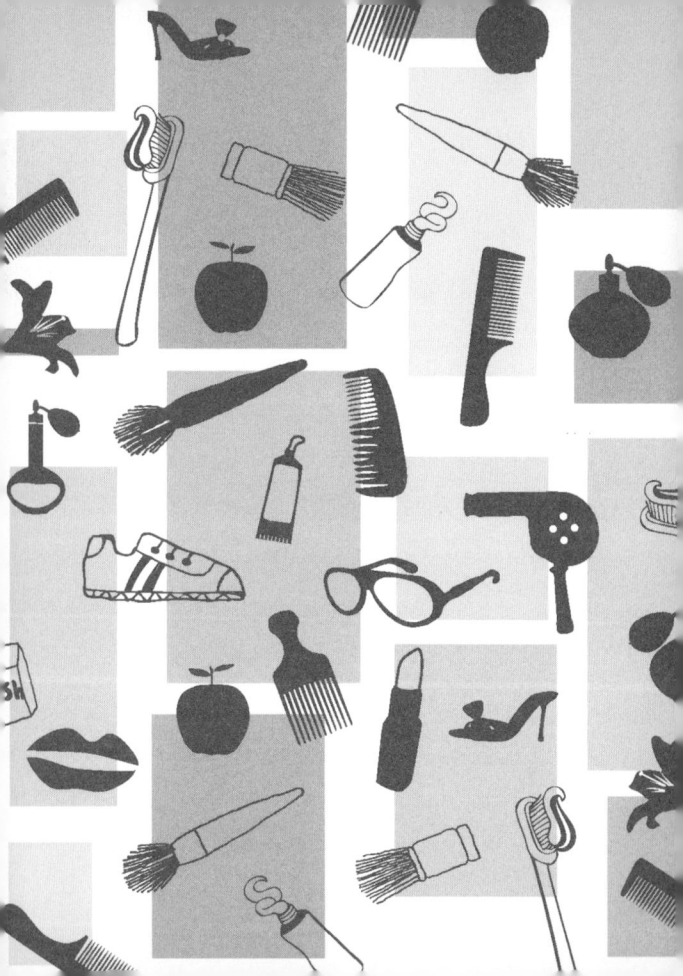

Kitchen cupboard
remedies

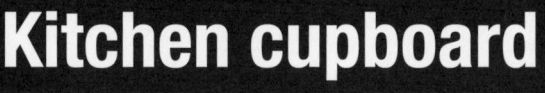

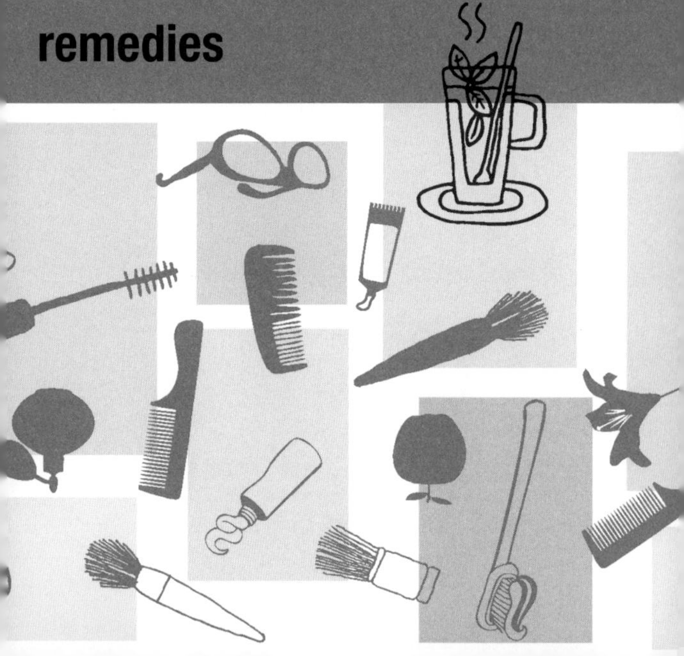

"I've heard that the ingredients in some deodorants can be carcinogenic. Is there a natural alternative?"

Mix ¼ cup of distilled witch hazel (cleansing and cooling) with ten drops of grapefruit-seed extract (fights odor-causing bacteria), 2 tablespoons of sage herbal extract, and ten drops of clary sage essential oil (an astringent). Pour into a spray bottle for an all-natural odor eater.

"How can I overcome strong body odor?"

Mix equal parts of apple cider vinegar and water together and slap it on before applying your usual deodorant.

"What can I do about my smelly feet?"

Make your own deodorizing talc by combining sandalwood and white oak bark powders and dusting it onto your feet each morning.

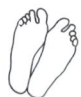

"How can I get smoother skin on my feet?"

Mash some strawberries and add them to a mixture of olive oil and sea salt. Soak your feet in warm water for 10 minutes, then rub your homemade scrub in circular movements across the feet before rinsing.

"How can I moisturize my dry feet?"

Mix one tablespoon of manuka honey into 2½ cups of almond or coconut milk and add it to a footbath.

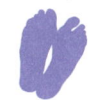

"How can I soothe my hard, dry feet?"

Add some milk or natural fruit juice to a footbath at the end of a long hard day. Both contain natural acids to help exfoliate the skin. Then use a pumice buffer to gently remove the dead skin cells.

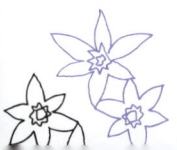

"How can I depuff my ankles?"

Soak some tea bags in boiling water, then add the tea to a footbath filled with more water and ice.

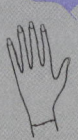

"My hands are dry and flaky. Is there a natural remedy?"

Mix a tablespoon of oats, a teaspoon of honey, five drops of almond oil, and 2 tablespoons of full-fat plain yogurt for a homemade moisturizing hand mask.

"How can I soothe my dry hands?"

Gently warm (not boil) a cup of full-fat milk, then soak your hands in it for 10 minutes. The lactic acid will act as an exfoliator to slough off dead skin cells.

"How can I give my hands a treat?"

Slather them in coconut oil and don some cotton gloves before bedtime. Rinse in the morning and you'll find yourself with silky smooth hands.

"How can I get smoother hands?"

Mix a tablespoon of white sugar with the juice of half a lemon and rub over the hands. The abrasiveness of the sugar particles removes dead skin cells while the acid in the lemon juice acts as a natural exfoliator.

"How can I prevent irritation on my hands?"

Detergents, soaps, and cosmetics frequently cause irritation and our hands get much of the battering. Add a few drops of tea tree oil to a bottle of rosewater and use this to wash your hands instead of traditional soap.

"How can I get a better night's sleep?"

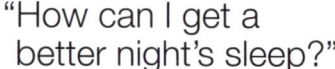

Put a few drops of marjoram oil in your bath at night. It's known for its soothing, sedative properties.

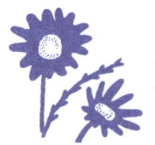

"What will make my bath more relaxing?"

Add a few drops of lavender oil and some coconut milk to your bath to ease your stress levels and soothe your skin at the same time.

"How can I make my own bath salts?"

Take an old sock and fill the foot with some sage and lavender leaves. Tie it up and let it float around your bath for a natural, chemical-free alternative.

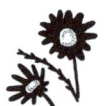

"Is there anything I can add to my bath to soothe my irritated skin?"

Ever since Cleopatra began bathing in milk, it has been used as a means of relaxing and nourishing the skin. Add 1¼ cups of full-fat milk to your bath to get the full benefits.

"Will bubble bath irritate my sensitive skin?"

Instead of using bought bubble bath, which may contain chemicals and other irritants, make your own. Add 20 drops of lavender oil to some baking soda and add to your bath as a soothing, fizzing mixture for your skin.

"Can I make an instant natural brightener for my skin?"

Mix equal amounts of olive oil and lemon juice and massage into your skin for five minutes.

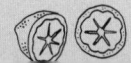

"What can I use on irritated skin?"

Licorice is known to soothe skin that has been irritated by an allergy. Chop up some natural licorice root, steep it in hot water overnight, then apply to the skin using a cotton ball.

"Can I soothe and exfoliate my skin at the same time?"

Mix yourself a homemade body scrub by combining 1 cup of full-fat plain yogurt (to soothe), with half a grated cucumber and 2 tablespoons of sea salt (to exfoliate). Rub onto dry skin before you get in the shower.

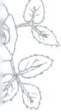

"How can I quench my dry skin?"

Follow an old Moroccan tradition and add a few drops of argan oil to some coconut or olive oil and spend three minutes massaging it into your face before bedtime.

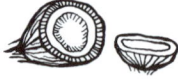

"Can I make my own soap for sensitive skin?"

Pour some ground oatmeal into the middle of a handkerchief and tie it at the corners to make a bundle. Use this to wash your skin: it's chemical-free and oats have healing properties.

"What's the gentlest way to exfoliate my skin?"

Mix your own moisturizing exfoliator by adding half a teaspoon of turmeric and a tablespoon of gram flour to 1⅓ cups of full-fat plain yogurt. Smooth a generous amount over your face, leave for ten minutes, and remove it using a muslin cloth.

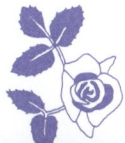

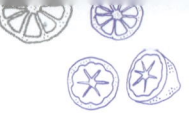

"How can I keep my face moisturized?"

Whip yourself up a mask by mashing the flesh of an avocado with a fork and adding a few drops of lemon juice. Smother it on, then use the pit to massage it in, using circular movement, before rinsing off.

"What's a natural way to combat the dry skin on my face?"

Combine a mashed banana with two tablespoons of full-fat plain yogurt. Apply a generous layer all over your face and leave on for ten minutes before rinsing thoroughly.

"Will tap water make my acne worse?"

It shouldn't, but if you want to treat your skin, stew some basil leaves in boiling water, leave it to cool, then place in the fridge overnight and splash this on your face first thing in the morning.

"*What home treatments can I do to lessen my acne?*"

Treat yourself to a homemade mask once a week by mixing some green clay (available from health food stores) and a few drops of rose geranium oil to help balance out the sebum and unclog your pores.

"Which natural oils are best for mature skin?"

Try grapeseed, apricot, myrrh, or pomegranate.

"*Can I cleanse my face with something chemical-free?*"

Some experts say that if you can't eat it, you shouldn't put it on your skin. So try splashing some cool almond milk (keep it in the refrigerator) on your face first thing in the morning and last thing at night.

"Can I make my own face exfoliator?"

Mash 1 cup of strawberries with two tablespoons of rice flour and massage onto dry skin for a few minutes before rinsing well.

"How can I give my skin the nutrients it needs?"

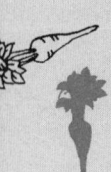

As well as eating a healthy diet, make a facemask by blitzing one avocado, one carrot, and one tablespoon of honey in a blender, applying it to your face, and leaving for ten minutes.

"Can I balance out my oily skin?"

Make a paste of baking soda and water and spread it evenly on your face. Leave it for 10 to 15 minutes, rinse and follow with a moisturizer for combination skin.

"How can I combat my skin's oily patches?"

Rub a slice of apple onto the areas twice a day, then splash with cool water.

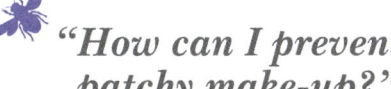

"How can I prevent patchy make-up?"

If your make-up starts sliding off certain parts of your face, it's most likely due to excess sebum in these areas. Before applying your make-up, dab a mixture of equal parts of lime juice and tea tree oil on the offending areas using a cotton ball.

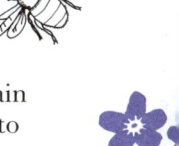

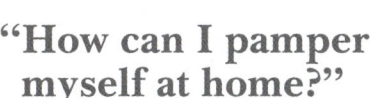

"How can I pamper myself at home?"

Try a mocha face mask by mixing four tablespoons each of finely ground coffee and cocoa powder, plus 1¾ cups of full-fat plain yogurt and half a teaspoon of manuka honey. Leave for 10 minutes before rinsing off.

"Can a bath help banish my wrinkles?"

Members of the Ancient Chinese Shang Dynasty (1600–1100 B.C.E.) believed in the rejuvenating power of herbal baths. Add some rose and elderflower petals plus a few drops of fennel oil and soak away your worries and wrinkles.

"How can I treat acne overnight?"

An ancient method from India is to mix a paste of equal quantities of sandalwood powder and turmeric, dab onto your acne and leave it on overnight.

"Is there a natural way to banish under-eye lines?"

According to ancient wisdom, an enzyme contained in papaya works like a natural acid to remove a layer of skin cells, so wrinkles appear less noticeable. Just mash it, apply, and leave for ten minutes.

"Does cucumber really help reduce under-eye puffiness?"

Cucumber does not contain a magic ingredient. When you're sleep deprived or have just had too many cocktails, dampen two teabags with cold water, then place them over your eyes for ten minutes. The cooling effect of the water and tannin in the bags acts as a natural astringent that restricts the blood vessels and tightens the skin's surface.

"How can I soothe red eyes after I've been crying?"

As tempting as it is to slather on eye creams, don't as they'll only increase the irritation. Instead, bathe your eyes in an eyewash from the pharmacy, then brew some camomile tea, add some ice and chill until it's really cold. Soak a couple of cotton balls in the tea then place over your eyes last thing at night before you go to sleep.

"How can I stop waking up with puffy eyes every morning?"

Raise the level of your head by sleeping with more than one pillow to prevent fluid retention around your eyes.

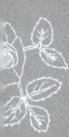

"How can I get radiant eyes without using chemicals?"

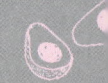

For centuries, members of the Mayan civilization have placed slices of avocado under the eyes to reduce puffiness and deliver essential fatty acids to the area.

"Is there anything in my kitchen I can use to remove eye make-up?"

Soak some cotton balls in warm water. Add a few drops of olive oil to the wet balls and use them to gently wipe your eyes.

"What can I use to perk up my under-eye area?"

Try massaging some almond oil very gently into the area every night before bed.

"Is there a natural way to treat cracked lips?"

Get kissable lips by mixing a teaspoon of moisturizing honey with a pinch of sugar to exfoliate the dead skin away. Rub gently over the skin's surface with a toothbrush.

"How can I keep my lips hydrated?"

Make yourself a homemade balm with a teaspoon each of honey and grated beeswax, ten drops of tea tree oil and five of lavender. The contents of a vitamin E capsule added into the mix is the magic ingredient.

"Is there anything I can use to moisturize my lips?"

Give your lips a deep moisturizing treatment by dabbing on castor oil last thing at night and let it be absorbed while you sleep.

"Can you suggest any natural toothpastes?"

Aloe Dent's Whitening Aloe Vera Toothpaste replaces the usual water in toothpastes with aloe vera and a blend of active ingredients to soothe the gums and protect against tooth decay. Green People also make natural pastes containing no fluoride, parabens, or sodium lauryl sulfate. Both can be found in most health food stores.

"Can I make my own mouthwash?"

Mix 1 cup of boiling water with six drops of peppermint oil (to freshen your breath) and half a teaspoon of myrrh tincture, which has potent disinfectant properties. Cool before using.

"What can I do to minimize plaque?"

Try eating a handful of cranberries after each meal. They reduce the stickiness of bacteria, preventing it from clinging to your teeth.

"How can I get bright, white teeth?"

Rub some bay leaves over the surface twice a week after normal brushing.

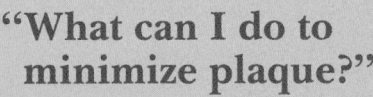

"How do I cure my brittle nails?"

Brittle means dehydrated. Apply a nail strengthener to protect them and massage hazelnut oil into your cuticles each day to restore them to health.

"Can I treat a fungal nail infection myself?"

Apply honey and leave it on for 15 minutes before removing. Do the same with garlic and alternate three times. Repeat the whole process twice daily until the infection clears up.

"How can I nourish my nails on a daily basis?"

Dip wet fingers in some cornmeal then massage it into your nails and cuticles.

"What can I do to add instant shine to my dull hair?"

Combine two tablespoons of ylang ylang and two of jasmine essential oils and apply while you're in the shower. Leave for a few minutes before rinsing off.

"Can I add an instant boost to dry, lackluster hair?"

Mix a tablespoon of olive oil, two of mayonnaise, and one egg then apply to your hair (avoiding the roots). Wrap in a warm towel, leave for 20 minutes, and rinse well three times.

"Is there a natural way to condition my dry hair?"

Try using palm nut oil every other wash instead of your usual conditioner. Avoid your roots because it may look flat otherwise.

"How can I rid my hair of product buildup?"

Rinse it in vinegar.

"How can I repair my hair after swimming?"

The result of being a water baby is dry, brittle hair. To repair the damage, mix one egg with two tablespoons of olive oil and leave it on your hair for ten minutes before rinsing.

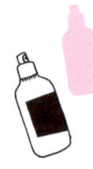

"How can I bring out the red in my hair?"

Apply a mixture of half carrot juice and half beetroot juice to damp hair. Wrap your head in a hot towel for 20 minutes before shampooing.

"How can I control my oily hair?"

Brew up an infusion of hot water and rosemary water and allow it to cool. After using, apply shampoo and conditioner as usual then give your hair a final rinse in the rosemary water.

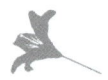

"How can I revive my dry, colored blonde hair?"

Whiz up a hair smoothie using a banana and a teaspoon of wheatgerm oil. Use it after shampooing, leave it on for ten minutes and rinse.

"How can I refresh my drab hair?"

This could be a sign of product buildup. Wash your hair in vodka to detox and bring back the shine.

"How can I add shine to my brown hair?"

Rinse it in black tea once every two weeks after washing.

"How can I stop burns from blistering?"

Soak a facecloth in a mixture of half vinegar and half water and apply to a mild burn. It will sting, but it will also not blister.

"Is there a natural way to combat canker sores?"

Brew a cup of camomile tea, leave it to cool, and swill around your mouth.

"How can I make my scars less noticeable?"

In Thailand, honey has traditionally been used to soften scar tissue and encourage the growth of new skin.

"Is there anything natural I can do to combat my hay fever?"

Inhale a few deep breaths of eucalyptus oil.

"How can I get rid of a blister?"

Avoid the temptation to pop it—you'll only spread the bacteria. Use a cotton swab to dab witch hazel on the offending blemish. It will dry it up and help the skin to heal naturally.

"How can I stop a burn from scarring?"

For a minor burn covering a small area, try dabbing a mixture of almond and lavender oil on to it to promote healing and prevent bacteria from colonizing the new skin.

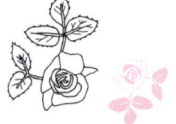

"How can I stop insect bites from itching?"

Cut a white onion in half and rub it gently on the bite. The natural sulfur will counteract the chemicals causing the itch.

"What's the best thing for insect stings?"

Use lemon juice and water on wasp stings and a mixture of baking soda and water on bee stings.

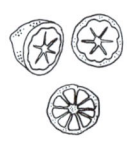

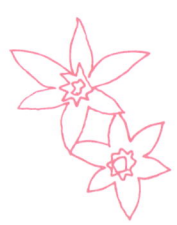

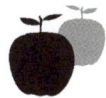

"Do I need lots of expensive supplements to boost my metabolism?"

Ditch the price-heavy pills and try good old apple cider vinegar, which has been used for centuries to boost metabolism. Make sure it's organic and cold pressed for the best results.

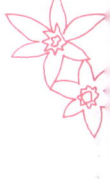

"What weird things do celebrities do to stick to their diets?"

Some Hollywood starlets are now hell bent on downing shots of vinegar before they eat to reduce their cravings and (they say) help the body digest food and flush out toxins.

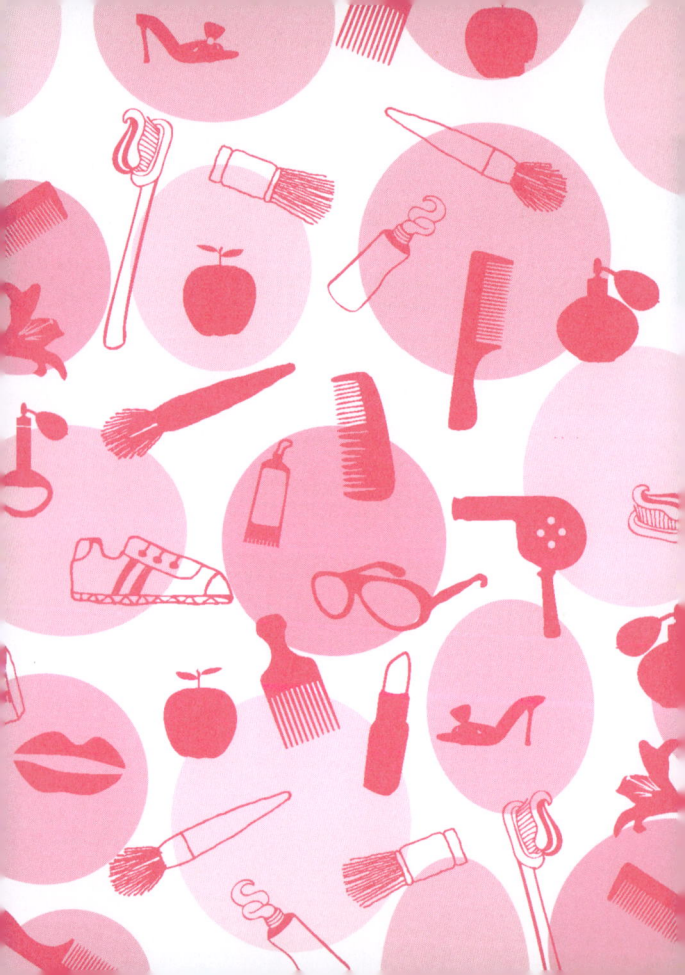

Alternative answers

"Should I take a multivitamin?"

A good multivitamin that contains a full spectrum of essential vitamins and minerals will support (not replace) a healthy diet. They come in pills, powders, and chewable tablets and Envida do a liquid version with a magnet at the bottom of the bottle. The magnet keeps the molecules in a bioactive state (it has an effect on living tissue), making it more effective.

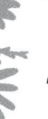

"What should I eat to get a good night's sleep?"

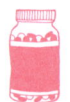

The old adage of a warm glass of milk really does help. Milk (like honey, turkey, and tuna) contains tryptophan, which is converted into serotonin, the body's sleep hormone.

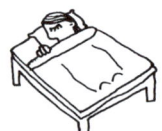

"How can I get the most from the fruit and vegetables I eat?"

Choose whole over ready-sliced fruit (which may have added preservatives to help keep its color) and eat the skin where possible (the concentration of antioxidants is highest in the skin of some fruit and vegetables). Eating seasonal, fresh, local produce will also help: the further your food has traveled, the more nutrients are likely to have been depleted.

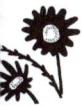

"Will giving up chocolate make me healthier?"

Chocolate contains tryptophan, a chemical that is converted to serotonin in the brain and lifts mood. Limiting your intake to a few squares a day and sticking to 70 percent cocoa solid dark chocolate will cut down the fats and sugars and give you a boost of antiaging antioxidants.

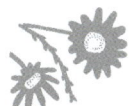

"How can I soothe an upset stomach?"

Make tea using one teaspoon of cinnamon and hot water. It will sooth your stomach, ease indigestion, and can even help settle diarrhea.

"What are the best foods for boosting energy?"

Skip the sugar-laden treats and go for a palmful of dried apricots or a banana with some nuts and seeds for a perfect balance of essential fats, protein, and carbohydrate to perk you up and keep you going for longer.

"Is all sugar bad for you?"

Steer clear of extrinsic sugars, found in cakes, candies and cookies, which include raw sugar, glucose, sucrose, or dextrose. Some natural (or intrinsic) sugars, including fructose, are found in fruits and vegetables and should be included as part of a healthy diet.

"How can I enjoy a drink and not blow my diet?"

If it's antiaging antioxidants you want, stick to red wine. But if you're watching your calories, make yours a vodka and low-calorie mixer or champagne.

"How can I beat bloating?"

The big bloat can happen as a result of a sluggish digestive system and constipation, so up your intake of insoluble fiber found in brown rice, couscous, seeds, and wholewheat breads.

"How do I know which are good fats?"

Omega-6 and omega-3 are essential fatty acids that keep your heart healthy, your skin radiant, your mind sharp, and your joints mobile. They are found in oily fish such as mackerel, salmon, and herring, plus nuts like brazils and walnuts.

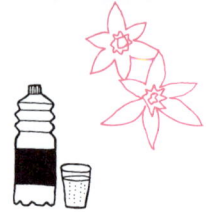

"Can drinking bottled water ever be eco-friendly?"

If you're concerned about the wastage of plastic bottles but don't want to compromise with tap water, Aquapax® water comes in a biodegradable paper carton made from sustainable resources.

"How can I fight wrinkles and treat myself when I eat out?"

Go for oysters: they're not only an aphrodisiac but they're also full of vitamin A, which helps slow down the aging process.

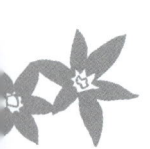
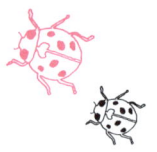

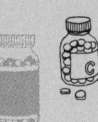

"How can I get a good range of vitamins and minerals?"

Learn to color-code foods. Orange and yellow foods (apricots, sweet potatoes, carrots, and squashes) are full of beta-carotene, which the body converts to antiaging vitamin A. Red foods (strawberries, raspberries, tomatoes, and red bell peppers) are full of vitamin C, which helps fight infection and absorbs iron more efficiently. Dark green foods (spinach, broccoli, kale, and cabbage) all contain iron, calcium, potassium, and folic acid, plus vitamins C, E, and K, and some of the B vitamins. They're basically nutritional powerhouses.

"What should I eat to burn fat?"

Coconut oil may technically be a fat, but Jennifer Aniston swears by it as a means of keeping herself trim. Some surveys have shown that it increases thyroid function and metabolism and helps you burn body fat.

"How do I know if I'm overweight?"

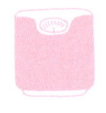

A good way to tell is the hip-to-waist ratio test. Divide your waist measurement at the narrowest part by the your hip measurement at the widest. Women with a ratio over 0.8 could benefit from losing weight.

"How can I stay wide awake all afternoon?"

To look and feel perky into the evening, ditch the carbs at lunchtime. Carbohydrates contain tryptophan, which is connected to the sleep hormone serotonin.

"How can I maintain my energy levels?"

Ensure you maximize the absorption of dietary iron by pairing it with a source of vitamin C. A glass of orange juice with your cereal, or some broccoli with a portion of red meat is a good way to start.

"What percentage body fat should I have?"

A healthy range for women is 22 to 25 percent. Some scales give a reading of your body fat percentage, but a professional fitness test will give a more accurate result.

"What's a nifty trick for weight loss?"

The new Lemon Juice Diet suggests that by squeezing lemon juice on your food, you increase the body's ability to break down food efficiently, which in turn may help you shed some pounds.

"How can I stop myself from grazing?"

Carry a toothbrush and some toothpaste, or chew sugar-free gum after each meal. It'll discourage you from eating more.

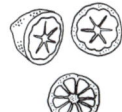

"How can I lose weight when I don't have time to cook healthy meals?"

Do what Jennifer Aniston does and get healthy, low-calorie, nutritionally balanced meals delivered to your door. There are web-based companies that deliver three meals and two snacks to your door each day and will even supply an extra meal or two if you have friends coming for dinner.

"Will I lose weight if I stick to ready-made, low-fat meals?"

Low-fat options often have added sugar to make them tastier. Always check the label to ensure there is no more than ¼ oz of total sugars per 4 oz of a product.

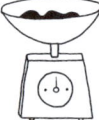

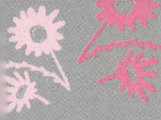

"What do celebrities do to stay slim?"

Victoria Beckham is reportedly a fan of Pur-erh tea from China. It claims to boost metabolism, stimulate digestion, reduce hunger, detox the blood, and strengthen the immune system. It is also supposed to help drinkers lose weight.

"How can I stave off the cravings between lunch and supper?"

Try including onions in your lunch. They contain chromium, a nutrient that helps keep blood sugar levels stable.

"Is there anything to help me keep my diet on track?"

DietPower is a spray based on natural ingredients such as honey and sea kelp, which helps balance metabolism, reduce food cravings, boost energy, and eliminate excess water retention so you don't feel so sluggish.

"How can I snack healthily?"

Do some clever snack swaps: oatcakes for cookies; unsalted, unsweetened popcorn for potato chips; a palmful of nuts and seeds for candies; two squares of dark chocolate for a bar of milk chocolate.

"How can I lose weight and get toned without bulking up?"

Try the new forms of dynamic or power Pilates, which combine the stomach-flattening and leg-honing movements of traditional Pilates with more aerobic activity to raise your heart rate and burn fat.

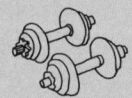

"What's a healthy snack that will boost my skin?"

Grab a handful of nuts or olives. Both are packed with essential fatty acids but contain less saturated (bad) fat than your average bag of potato chips.

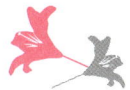

"What's a healthy snack that's good for my skin and hair?"

Grab a spirulina ball from a health food store. It's made from blue-green algae prized by the Mexican Aztecs and is believed to be one of the most nutrient-rich plant sources on earth. It contains antioxidants, phytonutrients, and probiotics, as well as vitamin E, zinc, vitamin B complex, and protein, which all promote healthy skin and hair.

"Which foods are highest in antioxidants?"

ORAC (oxygen radical absorption capacity) is a measure of the antioxidants in different foods. The acai berry has one of the highest ratings, followed by prunes, raisins, blueberries, raspberries, grapes, dark chocolate, kale, spinach, and broccoli.

"How can I look less tired?"

You may have an iron deficiency, so increase your consumption of green leafy vegetables, beef, and fortified cereals.

"What can I eat to reduce my stress levels?"

Reach for foods rich in vitamin B_6, such as bananas, sweet potatoes, and raisins, to help the body make serotonin, a brain chemical that gives you a calm, relaxed feeling.

"What will stop me feeling bloated after a meal?"

Eat some papaya at the beginning of a meal. It contains natural enzymes to help break down food.

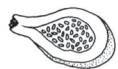

"Any tips for detoxing?"

It's the little things that count, so start each day with a cup of warm water with a slice of lime or lemon. It helps the body flush out toxins from the liver and gall bladder and may even help you lose weight.

"How can I detox in my own bathroom?"

Add some Epsom salts to your bath: these are known to help draw toxins from the skin.

"Is there anything other than fruit and vegetables that will help me detox?"

Try adding spices, such as turmeric, to your food: it improves digestion and helps eliminate toxins.

"What's the lazy girl's way to detox?"

Through your feet! Patch-it® is a system that involves placing sticky pads on the soles of your feet to stimulate circulation and draw out toxins while you sleep. It's worth it just to see your white-as-snow patch turn black and grimy overnight.

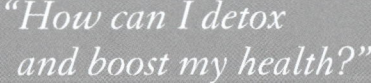

"How can I detox and boost my health?"

Get into wheatgrass shots. Drinking one serving is the equivalent of eating 2 lb of vegetables. It's full of antioxidants, helps cleanse the blood, boosts your energy, assists weight loss, and benefits everything from your teeth to your kidneys.

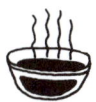

"I want to go on a detox but haven't the discipline to diet. Is there a way round it?"

The very idea of spending a week on nothing but celery juice leaves most people running for the chocolate. But if you're brave enough to try it, a coffee colonic irrigation carried out by a qualified colonic hydrotherapist uses caffeine to turbo-boost your liver and colon into releasing toxins, reducing excess water retention in your body and clearing your complexion.

"How can I ease a headache?"

Follow Ayurvedic medicine and massage sesame or almond oil into your scalp to release tension.

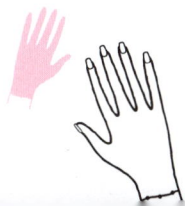

"My nose is permanently blocked but I don't have a cold. Is there anything I can do?"

A likely cause is dust mites found in your bed linen. Make sure you wash your sheets on a 94°F cycle (not less) to kill all of the dust mites.

"How can I clear a blocked nose?"

Pour boiling water over some rosemary, thyme and chopped lavender and inhale for a few minutes. Placing a towel over your head to catch the steam will intensify the treatment.

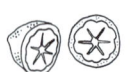

"How can I give myself a boost in the morning?"

Ditch your morning coffee (which plays havoc with your body's sugar levels) and use a deodorant containing lemon or eucalyptus oils, known to be uplifting and energizing.

"How can I avoid a hangover?"

Follow the five-step plan: Don't just drink, eat as well; and match each drink with a glass of water. Take milk thistle before drinking and when you go to bed. Take an electrolyte drink dissolved in some orange juice before bed to rehydrate and get a dose of vitamin C (it speeds up the metabolism of alcohol by the liver). Eat a banana when you wake up to restore potassium levels.

"How can I cure my body odor?"

As well as investing in a good antiperspirant, include more onions and garlic in your daily diet.

"How can I stop myself feeling light-headed in the bath?"

Try adding five tablespoons of salt to your bathwater.

"How can I soothe a sore throat?"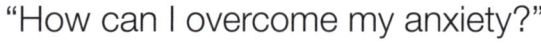

Try a cup of rosemary tea.

"How can I overcome my anxiety?"

Try valerian supplements, which have been found to relieve stress, worry, and insomnia.

"What will increase my energy?"

Bach flower remedies are 38 plant- and flower-based tinctures, each one used to treat a particular emotion or feeling. Olive Bach flower remedy is the one for tiredness and exhaustion, and a couple of drops taken daily in water can help boost flagging energy levels.

"Is there any effort-free way to tone up?"

If you don't fancy sweating it out on the treadmill, follow Madonna's lead and try a course of sessions on the Power Plate. It uses vibration to stimulate rapid muscle contraction, similar to the kind you get when weight training. You only have to stand on top of the plate in various positions, but the makers claim you can get the equivalent of a 30-minute workout in just 10 minutes.

"How can I boost my metabolism?"

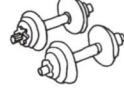

Do as the celebs do and add some weight training to your exercise regime. Far from bulking you up, it'll increase your resting metabolic rate, increase your muscle tone, and reduce your body fat.

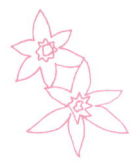

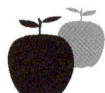

"How can I keep my metabolism revving?"

Rather than having three big meals a day, aim to eat five or six small meals and snacks a day and include some protein in each one.

"Any other tips for boosting metabolism?"

Make sure you always eat breakfast. This kick-starts your metabolism first thing in the morning and prevents the body from storing calories from fat when you do get around to eating lunch.

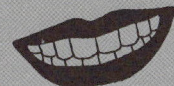

"How do celebrities keep their youthful looks?"

As well as surgery and some of the most expensive products money can buy, their secret weapon is beauty tonics. Kate Moss is a fan of Mangosteen Gold®, pure juice from the mangosteen fruit from Southeastern Asia. Makers claim it contains xanthones, powerful antioxidants that keep you looking young and even help you lose weight.

"How can I prevent a mid-afternoon energy slump?"

Make sure you always include protein in your lunch: it takes longer to digest, helps stabilize blood sugar levels, and makes you feel fuller for longer.

"How can I lift my mood in winter?"

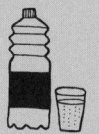

Exercise outdoors to get an invigorating blast of fresh air, up your vitamin D intake from the sun, and give your body a tougher workout than just pounding on the treadmill.

"How can I recover from flu fast?"

According to Ayurvedic medicine, a North American native root called goldenseal activates the white blood cells, which destroy viruses and bacteria. Supplements are available from health food stores.

"How can I find time to exercise?"

If you can't manage a full 30 minutes or an hour, do it in short bursts of ten minutes whenever you can. Studies show that the results can be just as effective as doing longer workouts less frequently.

"What do I need to start running?"

Your first priority should be a good pair of shoes. Have your feet scanned at a sports retailer to find out if you're a "pronator" (your ankles roll inward as you run), a "supinator" (your ankles roll outward), or a "neutral" runner (ankles right in the middle).

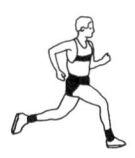

"Why aren't my crunches giving me a toned tummy?"

If you've got a layer of fat on your stomach, you could do three million crunches a day and still not see your abs. Unfortunately, you can't choose which areas you lose fat from so it's best to lose weight overall through cardiovascular and weight-bearing exercises to reveal that rock-hard tummy beneath.

"How can I get the most from my cardio workout?"

Instead of running, cycling, or swimming at a constant rate, vary it between faster and slower paces. Start by walking for three minutes and running for one, and repeating this for 20 minutes.

"Can you recommend a good low-impact exercise?"

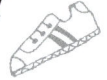
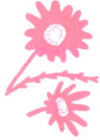

Aqua jogging has become all the rage for all those who want to tone up and burn calories using the resistance of the water without pressure on their joints. It involves wearing a buoyancy aid to keep you afloat in deep water while you *run* with weights attached to your wrists and ankles.

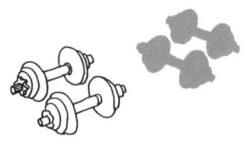

"Is there anything I can do to get rid of the rough bumps on the backs of my arms?"

"Chicken skin" syndrome is often caused by an omega-3 fatty acid deficiency in your diet. To do your new party dress justice, increase your intake of oily fish, such as salmon, and walnuts and seeds, which also help retain the skin's moisture for a healthy glow.

"Is there anything I can eat to stop me bruising so badly?"

Eat a diet rich in vitamin C and bioflavanoids found in berries, citrus fruits, and kiwifruit.

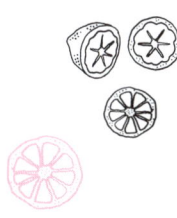

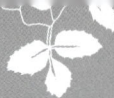

"How can I ease stiff muscles?"

Black pepper oil, or Piper nigrum, *is a warming, stimulating oil to soothe soreness when massaged into the skin. It's especially useful after exercise.*

"How can I make my back look great?"

With all the focus on abs, legs, and the bust, it's easy to forget our backs. Take up swimming or yoga to tone the muscles, then get a professional salon tan to even the skin tone with a healthy glow.

"What can I do about the fungal infections on my feet?"

Tea tree oil can help, but you should also go bare foot as often as possible. Keeping your feet penned up in hot, smelly runners will only increase your risk of infection.

"How can I keep my hands and feet warm in the winter?"

Try including more oily fish, garlic, and ginger in your diet to boost your circulation.

"How can I help shaving cuts heal quickly?"

Try rubbing the contents of a vitamin E capsule onto the cut.

"How can I make my bust look bigger?"

Short of implants, there's not a lot you can do. However, press-ups can help build up the pectoral muscle beneath the breast tissue, making your breasts seem bigger.

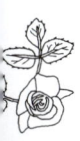

"How can I look good every day?"

Stop being so hard on yourself. There's nothing like self-criticism to make you seem less attractive than you really are.

"How can I make my nose look smaller?"

Avoid long hair—it will only make your nose more prominent. Go for mid-length or short styles and emphasize your best feature, whether it's a great jaw line or dazzling eyes.

"How can I look taller?"

Take some classes in the Alexander Technique. It focuses on balancing the body's neuro-muscular system by bringing about the natural movement through the head, neck, and back. It can improve posture, overall movement, breathing, and general health.

"Is there anything I can do to prevent stretch marks?"

To ward off those tell-tale silvery trails, keep your skin well moisturized with products containing vitamin E and cocoa butter. Also, eat plenty of flax, sunflower, sesame, and pumpkin seeds to boost your intake of essential fatty acids and zinc.

"How can I get a flat stomach for my party dress?"

Cut down on salt and sugar in the days before the party and sip peppermint tea between meals.

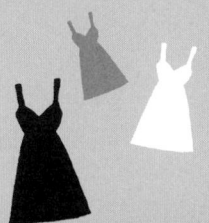

 ## "How can I stop my hands from getting dry?"

Make sure you dry them thoroughly after washing. Water left on the skin's surface will evaporate and leave them drier. Apply a nourishing hand cream after you have dried them.

"What's causing my eczema?"

Irritated skin is often caused by chemicals in cosmetics or household products, or sometimes a food intolerance. Common food allergens are dairy products, nuts, tomatoes, shellfish, and citrus fruits.

"I suffer from dermatitis. Is there anything I should avoid in my diet?"

Ditch the citrus fruits and lower your intake of saturated fats. A food allergy test can identify anything specific that may be aggravating the skin.

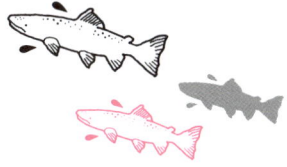

"Which are the best sources of skin-boosting omega-3 fats for a vegetarian?"

Flaxseeds, hemp seeds, and walnuts.

"What can I eat to improve my flaky skin?"

Ensure your diet includes plenty of essential fatty acids found in nuts, seeds. and oily fish. Adding oils, such as flaxseed or walnut, to your salads is another way of boosting your intake.

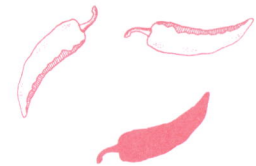

"What are the key nutrients for healthy skin?"

Your skin is the largest organ of the body and needs a wide variety of essential vitamins and minerals to stay healthy. The B vitamins (found in oily fish, poultry, and brown rice) are particularly important for repair and regeneration of skin tissue. Eating foods rich in vitamin C (kiwifruit, broccoli, bell peppers) will also help with the production of collagen and with wound healing.

"Is there anything I can eat to help my hard, dry skin?"

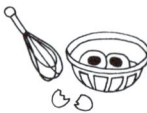

Up your intake of eggs, full-fat milk, carrots, mango, kale, and pumpkin, all rich in vitamin A.

"My eczema is ugly, itchy, and sore. How can I stop it from flaring up?"

Your doctor will give you a tube of steroid lotion that may rid you of your eczema, but will thin the skin making it more susceptible to bruising and stretch marks when used over a long period of time. A beauty editor's natural alternative is emu oil. Derived from the fat of an emu, it is rich in essential fats and linoleic acid and acts as a humectant, locking in moisture. Basting yourself in fat may not sound pretty, but it does work.

"What's a good natural healer for skin?"

Calendula oil has been used for centuries by healers for everything from acne and rosacea to eczema, bruises, spider veins, stretch marks, and wrinkles.

"How can I prevent cellulite?"

It can be genetic, but body brushing, getting regular exercise, avoiding too much sugar, saturated fat, and caffeine, not smoking, and drinking eight 8-oz glasses of water a day all helps.

"Is drinking the recommended eight 8-oz glasses of water a day necessary for healthy skin?"

While some experts say drinking this amount of water is needed to flush out the body's toxins and replace the moisture we lose daily in our breath, sweat, urine, and feces, others say that we can do this through drinking tea, coffee, and even fizzy drinks. In other words, the jury is still out, but water is better for your teeth and certainly won't do you any harm.

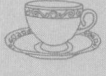 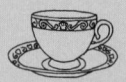

"What's an easy way to boost my skin?"

To get a double skin-boosting whammy, add a dressing of balsamic vinegar (rich in antiaging antioxidants) and olive oil (full of youth-saving essential fatty acids) to a healthy salad for lunch.

"What do I need for great skin and hair?"

Selenium is often referred to as the beauty mineral because it helps prevent premature aging and maintains healthy hair and skin. Eat three or four Brazil nuts a day to boost your intake.

"Is water aggravating my cellulite?"

While you're zealously getting your eight 8-oz glasses of water a day, you may be causing yourself more problems if it's fizzy. There are some experts who believe that aerated drinks, including soda water, encourage bloating and cellulite, so stick to still.

"What should I eat for radiant-looking skin?"

Try blueberries: they're packed full of skin-boosting vitamin C and antiaging antioxidants, and they're versatile too: sprinkle them on your morning cereal, blend them into a smoothie or grab a handful as a between-meal snack.

"Why does my jewelry make my skin red and irritated?"

You are probably having a reaction to the nickel. Paint a coat of clear nail polish onto your jewelry before wearing it to stop the reaction in its tracks.

"Is there anything I can take to protect my skin from environmental damage?"

A supplement of alpha lipoic acid (ALA) is said to protect against photo-aging of the skin.

"What's good for psoriasis?"

Try smoothing some cranberry oil onto the affected area last thing at night.

"What's the secret to smooth skin?"

Japanese women use silkworm cocoons, which contain a naturally woven silk protein called sericin. It helps balance the skin's amino acid content and exfoliates the dead skin cells, which can block pores, causing congestion and dry patches.

"How can I give my skin a boost in winter?"

Gotu kola (Indian pennywort) has been used for centuries in Indian and Chinese medicine and has been found to improve circulation, boost collagen production, and prevent oxidative damage, which leads to aging.

"What could be causing my dry skin?"

Any of the following could be contributing to the condition: central heating, air conditioning, excessively cold or hot weather, smoking, saunas, an allergic reaction, coffee, alcohol, or a poor diet lacking in essential fatty acids.

"What can I eat to help my acne?"

Acne occurs when the sebaceous glands in the skin produce too much sebum, blocking the pores and causing possible infection. Make sure you avoid sugar and saturated fats and eat a diet rich in zinc from foods like shellfish, turkey, and brown rice.

"How can I make my skin less puffy?"

Puffiness is often caused by water retention. Skip the fizzy drinks, which act as a diuretic but also leach bones of essential potassium, and go for nettle, dandelion, and juniper teas.

"Can natural oils actually help oily skin?"

Grapefruit, yarrow, and rosemary essential oils are all natural astringents to cleanse the skin. Tea tree, lavender, and rosewood oils have all been known to help acne, while peppermint and lemongrass can lessen blackheads.

"How can I heal my acne scars?"

Supermodel Jasmine Guinness relies on a South American face oil, Rosa Mosqueta, which can be used on the face and body to heal scars and even improve the appearance of stretch marks.

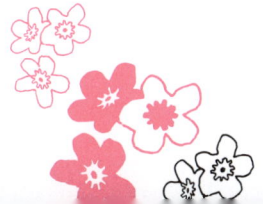

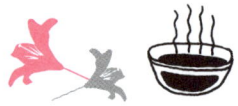

"Is there anything I should avoid if I've got broken capillaries on my face?"

Don't expose your face to very hot water or steam (so no saunas), harsh exfoliators, or too much alcohol or sunbathing. Natural, chemical-free products and make-up would also be a good investment because they're less likely to irritate your skin further.

"Are there any natural ways to ease acne?"

According to Chinese medicine, acne is a result of too much heat: your skin is literally like a volcano waiting to erupt. Try burdock, dandelion, and red clover teas to help purify the liver and blood, leaving the liver free to deal with hormones efficiently and minimize the risk of breakouts.

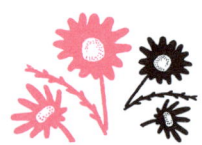

"Is there anything I should avoid diet-wise if I suffer from acne?"

Reduce your intake of salty foods and those rich in iodine (like shrimp and seaweeds), which stimulate oil production. Replace them with fruit and vegetables containing beta-carotene, such as tomatoes, carrots, and squashes.

"Is there a noninvasive way to banish wrinkles?"

Safetox® is a device worn around the head that delivers electronic pulses. It inhibits the muscles that cause wrinkles and stimulates those that lift the face. You use it for five minutes every day until you see results, then maintain with a session three times a week.

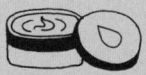

"How can my diet help me ward off wrinkles?"

Get your wholegrains. Foods such as wheat, oatmeal, and brown rice all contain zinc, which helps maintain the elastin fibers in collagen.

"How can I prevent breakouts after having my eyebrows threaded?"

Swipe a cotton ball drenched in witch hazel over your brows and forehead.

"Will putting olive oil on my skin make it more radiant?"

The benefits of olive oil are well known. However, if you really want to give your skin a zing, the sap from the olive leaf (rather than fruit) is said to contain up to 40 times more youth-boosting antioxidant polyphenols.

"Which oil really works on oily skin?"

Bergamot oil has been used for centuries for its antiseptic and healing properties, making it perfect for people with acne, infected skin, or even minor wounds.

"What soothes a rash?"

According to ancient Ayurvedic medicine, rashes must be treated from the inside as well as the outside of the body by drinking a cup of fresh coriander tea each night.

"How can I clear congested pores?"

Make a facial steambath by adding a few drops of peppermint oil to a bowl of hot water to cleanse and tighten your pores.

"How can I combat blackheads naturally?"

As odd as it sounds, applying mandarin oil helps refine the skin.

"How can I get rid of severe facial hair?"

If threading or tweezing won't do, Vaniqa® is a prescription drug that works by dissolving the hair follicle.

"What can I eat to keep my eyes healthy as I age?"

Make sure you get enough lutein, which is found in carrots, broccoli, spinach, Brussels sprouts, and kale.

"Why is it that no matter how much sleep I have, I still have under-eye circles?"

These shadows often run in families or may be caused by nasal congestion. When your nose is blocked, the veins that usually drain down from your eyes to your nose get wider and darker, causing the discoloration.

"How can I make plucking my eyebrows less painful?"

Try smoothing canker sore gel on first, then leaving it for a few minutes before you begin plucking.

"How can I brighten my bloodshot eyes?"

Soak some cotton balls in milk and apply them to the eyes for ten minutes while you relax.

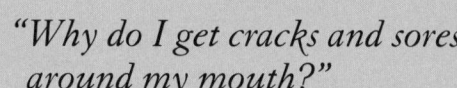

"Why do I get cracks and sores around my mouth?"

You may have a vitamin B deficiency. Make sure you eat plenty of brown rice, poultry, and oily fish, as well as chicken livers.

"How can I make my teeth less sensitive?"

Look for a natural toothpaste and mouthwash containing tea tree (a natural antibacterial ingredient), cloves, or perilla seed extract. Cloves have been used for centuries to soothe toothaches and perilla promotes healthy teeth and gums.

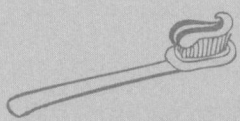

"What should I eat to keep my teeth healthy?"

Magnesium and calcium are the two most important nutrients that work in tandem to give you strong, healthy teeth. Eat plenty of magnesium-rich nuts, seeds, leafy green vegetables, and salmon. Eat dried apricots and dairy produce for calcium.

"How can I reduce my smile lines without surgery?"

Consider a dental facelift, which replaces any missing teeth and aligns others into their correct position in order to support the jaw and tighten the muscles and skin around the mouth, and strengthen the bones.

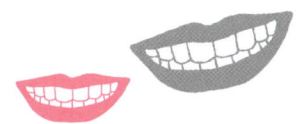

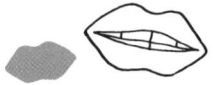

"Does the acid in fruit harm my teeth?"

Instead of reaching for acidic fruits like oranges, choose strawberries, which are kinder on tooth enamel but are still packed with vital vitamin C, essential for both healthy teeth and gums.

"What will soothe my toothache?"

Apply a few drops of clove oil to the aching area of the gum.

"Is there anything I could eat to combat my dry hair?"

If your locks are looking a little strawlike, try upping your intake of vitamin A, found in carrots, dark green leafy vegetables, sweet potatoes, and apricots.

"What on earth is "bubble hair"?"

It is when an overly hot hairdryer softens the protein in the hair shaft and causes water trapped within it to boil, forming tiny bubbles of steam.

"Why is my hair drier in the winter?"

You'd think that the lack of sun would make hair less vulnerable to dryness. But switching from your central-heated house to the Arctic temperatures outside causes your hair to alternate between dry and frizzy, and damp and lank. Make yourself a winter hair reviver tonic using three tablespoons of vodka and one of witch hazel. Rub it in your palms then massage into your scalp for five minutes before rinsing.

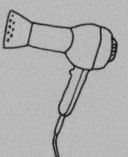
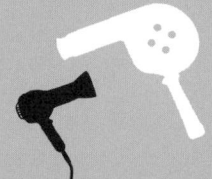

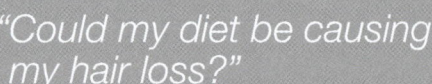

"Could my diet be causing my hair loss?"

Hair loss occurs as a result of many things, age, genes and certain medical and scalp conditions included, but may also be a sign of zinc deficiency. Increase your intake of seafood, poultry, eggs, grains, and legumes to boost your zinc levels.

"What's the best way to treat dandruff?"

A normal, healthy scalp sheds small flakes of skin as part of its cell regeneration process. Dandruff is caused by a fungus called Malassezie, which can both speed up shedding of the skin and cause larger, more noticeable flakes. To treat it, look for shampoos with herbs such as willow extract to exfoliate the skin and fenugreek to soothe the irritation. Shampoos with a base of castor and coconut oils will also help nourish the scalp and remove impurities.

"Are there any supplements I can take for my hair?"

To keep your locks glossy, try silica or horsetail.

"My hair is looking distinctly lackluster. How can I put some life back into it?"

Poor hair condition can indicate nutritional deficiencies. Adding flaxseed oil to salads should restore you to your former glossy-locked glory within weeks.

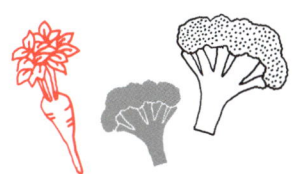

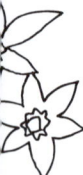

"How come whichever products I use, I still have dry, brittle hair?"

If you've tried anything and everything to smooth your troubled locks, it may be the water in your bath or shower that's responsible. Find out if you are in a hard water area (soft water makes soap froth more easily, whereas hard water does not) and get a filter fitted if you are.

"How can I make my hair look thicker?"

Adding layers can create the appearance of more volume, while highlights or lowlights provide texture for a fuller, thicker look.

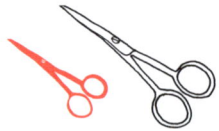

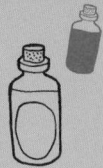

"How can I change my hairstyle without losing the length?"

Consider having layers cut into your length, adding highlights or lowlights, a full color change, or even bangs. If that's all too drastic, changing your parting from the side to the middle (or creating a zigzag) can alter your look dramatically.

"What's a good haircut to complement an older face?"

Traditionally, women of a certain age have been advised against having long hair, but if it's healthy and strong, flaunt it. Just avoid anything with sharp lines or asymmetric that will be too severe. Feathered layers that frame and soften your face will take years off you.

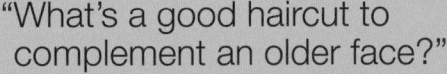

"How can I stop my hair from thinning?"

Hair loss can be down to genetics, stress, nutritional deficiencies, and other lifestyle factors, not least smoking. Researchers have found that smokers are more likely to suffer from premature hair loss and early graying, so stub it out and keep your hair on.

"When's the best time of year to get highlights?"

Traditionally women have gone lighter in the summer and toned down their highlights for the winter. Consider going fairer in winter to lift rather than drain your skin when it's at its palest.

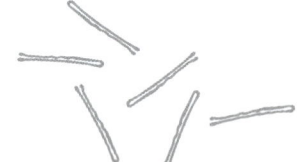

"Why does my hair keep breaking?"

It could be that you're causing breakages by brushing your hair when it's wet. Use a wide-toothed comb instead of a brush on wet hair and be gentle with your hair. A detangling spray will also stop you yanking at it furiously.

"How long should I wait before going all-over gray?"

You should be at least 40 percent gray before you consider the all-over look. Before then, go lighter with some highlights to lift your hair color.

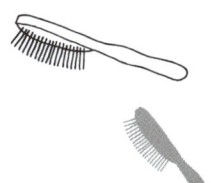

"What's the best way to blow-dry frizz-prone hair?"

Always use a dryer with a diffuser, which emits heat evenly and with less intensity, making your hair less liable to get dry, brittle and frizzy.

"What type of bangs will suit me?"

Side bangs suits a round face, feathered or choppy bangs suit a square face, while full, blunt bangs work on a long face.

"How can I use my hair to look younger?"

Open your face up by tying your hair back or pinning some of the front sections back.

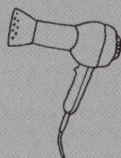

"Is there anything I can take to prevent hair loss?"

Saw palmetto berry supplements have been used to block the formation of hair follicle-killing dehydrotesterone and promote thick, healthy locks.

"How can I prepare myself for a dramatic haircut?"

Visit www.thehairstyler.com, where you can upload a picture of yourself then try out some different styles.

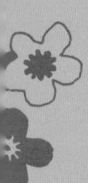
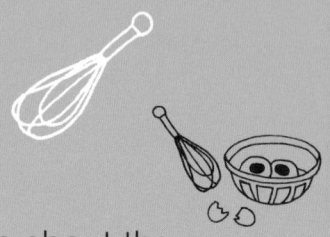

"What can I do about the ridges on my nails?"

You could have a zinc deficiency so invest in a good supplement, up your intake of oysters, almonds, haddock, and eggs and buff your nails daily to even out their surface.

"Will eating more dairy products stop the white spots in my nails?"

It's one of the great beauty myths that those spots are a sure sign of a calcium deficiency. Instead, try taking a zinc supplement.

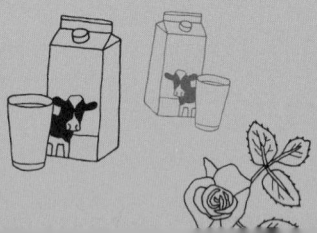

"Is there anything I can take to strengthen my nails?"

Biotin supplementation has been found to improve the appearance of hair and nails.

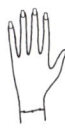

"How can I make my nails grow faster?"

Fingernails grow faster than toenails, and the rate relies on them receiving a good supply of blood. A Ginkgo biloba supplement can improve circulation in your hands and stimulate your stubby nails.

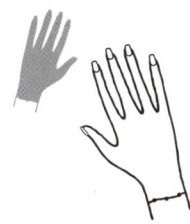

Dress to impress

"How can I add interest to my wardrobe?"

Aside from trying out new colors and adding to your collection of accessories, experiment with different textures. Mix a rope necklace with a neoprene (synthetic rubber) top, or a tulle skirt and silk blouse, and throw out the old rules about playing it safe.

"What should I wear to the gym?"

Your old jogging pants and a T-shirt will leave you feeling demoralized and sweaty. Today's sportswear ranges are specially designed to keep you sweat-patch free and make you look good. The right kit can also help prevent injuries and stop you from giving up after a couple of weeks. The right running shoes are essential, so have your feet scanned at a sports shoe store.

"What are the mainstays of a good wardrobe?"

Every women needs...

- A pair of black jeans
- A white shirt
- Some simple, fitted T-shirts
- A pair of comfortable high heels
- A pair of ballet pumps
- A large leather purse
- A classic trench coat
- A fitted blazer
- A little black dress

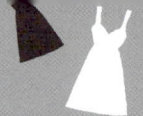

"How do I buy vintage?"

Follow the three golden rules. Quality: are there any rips, tears, or marks on it? Style: it may be vintage but does it still look modern? You don't want to look like you're wearing fancy dress. Wearability: is it part of an overall look that you know suits you? Don't step too far out of your own boundaries; you need to feel comfortable wearing it.

"If I'm going to splash out on one item, what should it be?"

Go for broke with some designer shoes. You won't grow out of them if you put on weight and they're less vulnerable to the fickle ways of fashion.

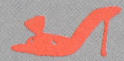

"What are the best tactics for sale shopping?"

So many action plans suggest tiresome lists before you shop, but staying sale savvy will mean that you can afford to be more flexible.

- Have a total budget and stick to it.
- Don't buy trends. Buy classics that suit your body shape and will still look good in years to come.
- Arrive early and get your elbows out: competition can be fierce.
- Check the returns or exchange policy.
- Ask yourself whether it's really a bargain or if you're buying it because the label says it's at a discounted rate.

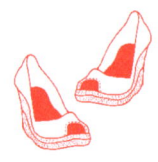

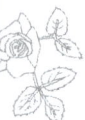

"How do I get celebrity style for less?"

If you're on a budget but want high style, www.asos.com has more affordable versions of the clothes celebrities having been snapped wearing.

"How can I re-vamp my wardrobe on a budget?"

Forget the stores. The latest craze for those who want to be ethical and update their wardrobes on a budget is clothes swapping, or "swishing" parties. Visit www.swishing.org for tips on how to host your own.

"How do I find designer clothes at bargain prices?"

Look for designer sales: there are websites that send you alerts about up-and-coming sales and sample sales, or try websites such as www.koodos.com, which have permanently discounted items.

"How can I revive last year's wardrobe?"

Start by caring for your current items. At the beginning of each season, make a mental note to have your coat dry-cleaned, your best shoes reheeled, and your knitwear de-fluffed.

"How can I avoid looking frumpy during pregnancy?"

The empire line is your godsend. Dresses and tops in this style will nip you in beneath your blossoming bosom and skim over your belly.

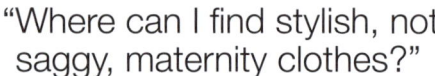

"Where can I find stylish, not saggy, maternity clothes?"

Mama-la-mode.com is an online boutique featuring maternity collections from over 60 designers who rate style and comfort as being of equal importance. Outfits even come with a trimester rating to tell you at which stage in your pregnancy they will be most suitable.

"How can I find my style?"

Experiment with clothes from different designers and shops to know which suit your shape and style best. Are you preppy in Ralph Lauren, glamorous in Valentino, on-trend in Marc Jacobs, or cute in Luella?

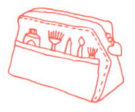

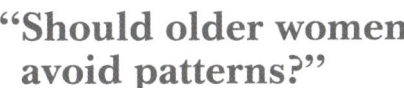

"Should older women avoid patterns?"

Use pattern and color to highlight your best assets and let darker colors make your problem areas melt into the background.

"Can anyone get away with neutral colors?"

The trick is to find a tone that suits you. If your skin is on the dull/gray side, warm it with very pale pinks and nudes. Taupes and fawns can look good on yellowish skins and white skins can work pinks or creams.

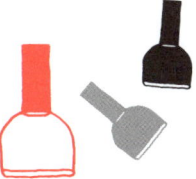

"What's the difference between black and white tie?"

Black tie is formal and white tie is even more so. For the former, men should wear tuxedos and black bow ties, and tail coats with white bow ties for the latter. There's less of a difference for women, but floor-length gowns are the norm for white tie, while shorter or prom-style dresses may be acceptable for black tie.

"How do you pull off bright colors?"

If you're stuck in a black wardrobe hole, bright colors can actually make you look younger and slimmer. Instead of going head-to-toe bright, wear a vibrant color on your top or bottom, whichever you consider to be your best asset.

DRESS TO IMPRESS

"Is black and navy always a no-no?"

The old fashion rulebook has been thrown out of the window, so mix black and navy for a smart look, try pink and red for something bright and breezy, and make your own color combinations according to what suits you.

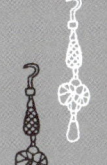

"How do you find knitwear that suits you?"

Slimmer types can afford to go chunky with cable knits and jumper dresses. If you're fuller-figured, go lighter with wool and stretch mixes, and fitted cashmere jumpers or cardigans.

"What type of top will make my bust look bigger?"

Pick sleeveless tops and halternecks.

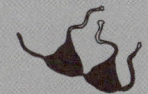

"Can anyone wear turtlenecks?"

Big-bosomed ladies should steer clear and opt for more flattering V-neck sweaters instead.

"How do celebrities stay sweat-patch free on the red carpet?"

Those in the know use a Drysol antiperspirant, which is applied at night for two or three days before a big event and can stop sweating almost completely.

"Which fabrics are best for minimizing sweat patches?"

Stick to natural materials such as silk, linen, and cotton and avoid the nylons and polyesters—a recipe for sweat-patch disaster.

"Does black really suit everyone?"

Black can be draining when worn next to older skins. Instead of navy (very matronly), look for shades of brown, taupe, and fawn to flatter your skin tone and bring warmth to your face.

"Which perfume should I wear when?"

Traditionally, light floral or citrus scents have been worn in the day while deeper, musky or vanilla-based fragrances pep up an evening party look.

"What's the best way to keep zips from breaking?"

Run beeswax over them to keep them working smoothly so you don't need to yank at them.

"What's the best way to store clothes?"

Hanging allows clothes to be aired. Choose wooden hangers over wire or plastic ones to help them keep their shape.

"What's the best way to care for cashmere?"

Hand, rather than machine, washing goes without saying. There are now cashmere shampoos that allow you to treat your best woolies with the same degree of expert care that you would your own hair.

"How do you stop new knitwear from shedding hair all over your other clothes?"

Pop it in the freezer for an hour when you first buy it.

"How do you dress for a day wedding with an evening reception?"

The secret is in the coverup. Wear a glam knee-length or just-above-the-knee dress (anything shorter is a bit risqué, anything longer a bit frumpy) with thin straps or some kind of shimmer detailing. Sling on a cool linen jacket for summer daytime weddings and a faux fur stole for winter ones.

"Can you wear white to a wedding when you're not the bride?"

Almost anything goes at most weddings nowadays. However, to avoid getting death stares from the bride, opt for cool tones of very pale yellow, ice blue or pink, which are off-white rather than pure, wedding-gown white.

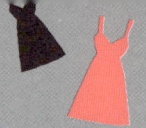

"When it comes to party dresses: no straps, straps, or sleeves?"

Strapless dresses have been done to death, but the choice should ultimately rest on the shape of your shoulders. Broad shoulders should pick narrow straps, while narrow shoulders can go for full or cap sleeves. If you've got particularly honed, square shoulders, strapless will work but it should never be attempted by those who have rounded or sloping ones.

"Is a wrap dress really a fail-safe for every woman's wardrobe?"

Forget the hype about wrap dresses: if you've got a boyish figure, it's only going to make your lack of curves more obvious.

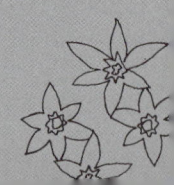

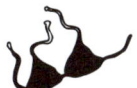

"Which bra should I wear under a backless dress?"

Look for brands that do stick-on support. Bras come with an adhesive strip to attach to your skin so there are no unsightly straps.

"What kind of dress will add curves to my boyish frame?"

Get a gown that's cut on the bias to create the illusion of having bigger hips.

"What's the perfect party dress for broad shoulders?"

Go glam in a dress that clings to your waist then has a bit of a kick to the skirt to balance out the breadth of your shoulders.

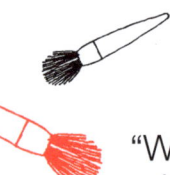

"What's the best dress style to hide a tummy?"

Look for plunging V-necks that accentuate your breasts. An empire-line dress will nip you in just beneath your breasts then skim over, rather than cling to, your tummy.

"Are there any dress styles that will make my bust look bigger?"

Boost your top half by choosing a dress with ruffles or a bust-lifting bodice that will also narrow your waist by comparison.

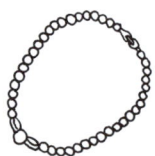

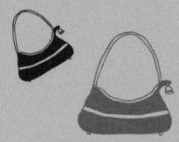

"Can women over 50 really not wear mini-skirts?"

Let not your age be your guideline, but your legs. Regardless of current trends or so-called 'fashion age-limits', you should always dress for your own body. If your legs are your best feature, show them off whatever your age. Just keep it to mid-thigh and no shorter if you are older to avoid comments about mutton *and* lamb.

"What's the best style of skirt to make my legs look longer?"

If your legs are shorter than you'd like them to be, always opt for the good old mini. The more of your legs on show, the longer they'll look.

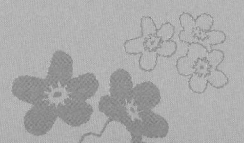

"What are the best leg-lengthening slacks for shorter women?"

Straight-legged, flat-fronted pants with the hem skimming the ground. Tucking your top into your pants will also shorten your torso and elongate your legs by comparison.

"What type of slacks will make my bum look smaller?"

Go for dark colors, no back pockets and low-rise styles to streamline your behind.

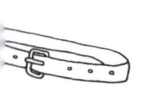

"What type of jeans suit a pear shape?"

Ditch the skinny jeans that taper at the ankle (and emphasize your hips), and go for straight legs or boot cuts, ensuring they reach almost to the ground when you're wearing heels. Darker washes will all slim your legs.

"How do I find jeans to fit my slim frame?"

Go for a denim-stretch mix, which will cling to rather than wrinkle away from your legs. Always do the acid test: do they sag at the back?" A pair with pockets at the back will beef up a nonexistent bum.

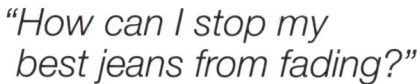

"How can I stop my best jeans from fading?"

Minimize the frequency of washes, turn them inside out, and always use a cool wash. If things get really bad, you can always try a color wash to replace some of the dye, though this is best kept for black jeans.

"What style of jeans will flatter my big hips?"

Wide-legged or flared styles will balance out your hips. Make sure they're flat-fronted with no extra pockets because these tend to add bulk.

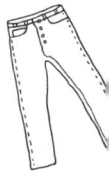

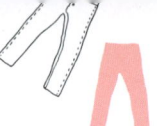

"What's the best color for jeans?"

It used to be stonewashed, then black or faded gray skinnies were all the rage. Black and white will always be classic, but there are now jeans in bright colors that are a good addition to any wardrobe.

"Jackets open or done up? What's more slimming?"

Skinny minnies can afford to button up, but if you want to slim down, go for one size smaller than you normally would and wear it open over a dark-colored top. Avoid bulky zips or pockets—they'll only make you look boxy.

"How can I stop jackets from making me look boxy?"

Avoid the cube look and buy a single-buttoned jacket, which accentuates your waist and adds shape to your body.

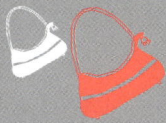

"Single- or double-breasted?"

If you're small up top, a double-breasted coat or jacket will give you shape. Anyone with a large bust should stick to single-breasted or even single-buttoned versions to avoid looking larger than they really are.

"How do pear shapes get away with wearing jackets?"

Never go for anything cropped or that rests just above your bottom and hips—you'll only make them look wider. Opt for longer-length jackets that cover your bum, and wear dark colors on your bottom half.

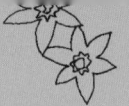

"How do you buy a winter coat?"

Buy early: it may seem odd to buy a coat in August, but the best ones sell out fast. Try it on with shoes that you'll wear in winter and go for detail—big buttons, over-sized collars, pockets, and cuffs make the difference between an outstanding coat and an ordinary one. Pick classic shapes and you can afford to make a big statement with color: red always looks good on dull winter days.

"What's the best style of bikini to suit my petite frame?"

Traditional advice would have you wear high-cut bottoms, but this can overemphasize your thighs. Stick to halternecks to give you shape up top, and boy shorts to broaden your narrow hips.

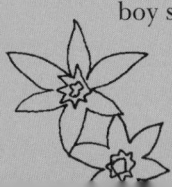

"How can I make bikini buying more bearable?"

Don't ruin your self-confidence by trying on swimwear under the harsh lights of a changing room: buy over the Internet. That way you can buy multiple sizes of the same design and several different styles, try them on in the comfort (and nice lighting) of your own home and send them back if necessary.

"How can I find a swimsuit to flatter my shape?"

If you're feeling the pressure to look good on the beach, invest in a tailormade swimsuit. Many stores are now offering a personalized fitting service and will make a swimsuit to the color and design of your choice.

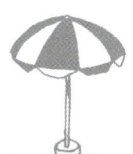
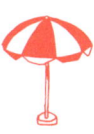
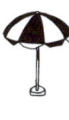

"What kind of swimsuit flatters bigger-bellied women?"

Ditch the bikini and traditional bathing suit and go for a tankini. The longer top should skim the top of your swimming briefs and hide your problem area.

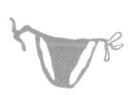

"What's the best bikini for busty types?"

Take a tip from curvy celebs like Kelly Brook, who look great in halterneck bikinis. Ironically, the key here is coverage, so avoid string bikinis and prevent yourself looking bigger by ditching the horizontal stripes.

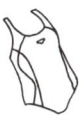

"Can I get the coverage of a one-piece bathing suit and still show a bit of flesh?"

Go for a clever stencil-like effect with a cut-out swimsuit that provides the coverage of a traditional bathing suit but has holes in unusual places such as the hip, back, or shoulder.

"How can I look taller during the swimsuit season?"

Pick swimsuits or bikinis with diagonal stripes.

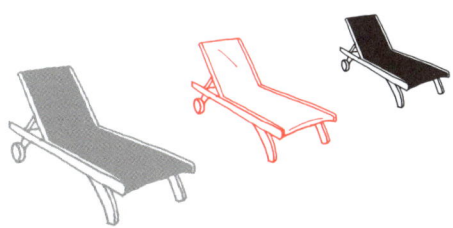

"Is there a bra that will work on all occasions?"

Bras are the new accessories and buying several is an absolute must. To cover the essentials, invest in the following:

An everyday bra: pretty enough to make you feel good but not overly fussy. It must fit perfectly.

A sports bra: to support and keep everything where it should be while you're at the gym or jogging.

A T-shirt bra: seamless and smooth.

A multiway: for tricky dresses and tops.

A visible bra: one that you'll be proud to show just a hint of on a night out.

"What style of bra will make my bosom look bigger?"

Go for a half-cup plunge with a bit of extra padding. The angle of the cups gives the illusion of your breasts being fuller than they really are.

"How can I stop my panty hose from snagging in the wash?"

Put them inside a pillowcase.

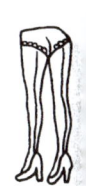

"Are sheer panty hose ever okay?"

Sheer panty hose are really only acceptable for the office. Go for opaque black (you can even get away with this during cool summers) or bare legs. If you really must have sheer, go for some wellfitting panty hose with sheen.

"How do you get away with patterned panty hose?"

You can't. Patterned panty hose are the equivalent of novelty socks, ties, and boxers on men. If you're bored of your old navy and black ones, go for a bright color or gray. Alternatively, change the texture and go for ribbed panty hose.

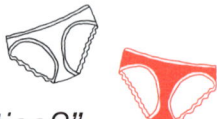

"Thongs or panties?"

Thongs have their place (under white jeans, tight slacks, or clingy dresses to prevent VPL), which doesn't include poking out above your jeans. If you're going to flash some pant, better make it some vintage-style French panties or boy shorts in bright colors or polka dot prints, plus quirky (rather than tacky) lace detailing.

"How can I stop my underwear from being ruined in the wash?"

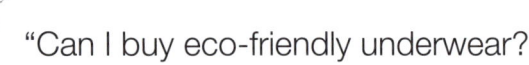

Graying panties, limp bras, and wonky underwiring are no basis for an elegant look. Try washing your undies inside a laundry bag to prolong their shelf life.

"Can I buy eco-friendly underwear?"

If you've jumped on the green bandwagon, look for labels such as Green Knickers.

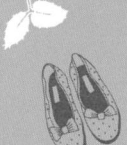
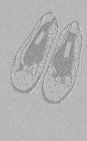

"Will ballet pumps suit me?"

There's a pump to suit everyone, but it's all in the toe. If you have largish feet, a fully rounded toe will make them seem smaller. If you've got ballerina's feet, squarer or more oval toes will look good. Anyone can get away with a bit of toe cleavage (when the crack in your toes is just showing).

"How do you walk in high heels?"

The rules are: keep your head up and shoulders back, take small steps rather than big strides, and try to keep the weight back on your heels. In reality, it's all about practice.

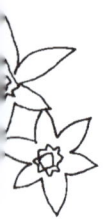

"How can I find knee-high boots to fit my chunky calves?"

Try www.thebootmakers.com, who specialize in boots to fit both slim and wider calves.

"Can you wear tights with open-toed shoes?"

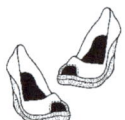

No, never, no. You can (just about) get away with some brightly colored ankle socks and open toes if you're going for a young, edgy look.

"I love heels, but how can I look stylish in flats?"

Go for simple ballet pumps, riding boots, or classic Converse runners.

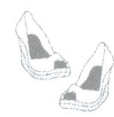
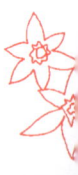

"Ankle boots or knee-highs?"

If you've got legs like a gazelle, you can wear ankle boots with everything from leggings to skinny jeans or mini skirts. They should be avoided by anyone with short legs because they create a cut-off at the ankle, making you look stumpy.

"How can I keep my shoes in top condition?"

Instead of bundling your trillions of pairs one on top of another to fester at the bottom of your wardrobe, invest in some special shoes boxes, such as transparent boxes that open at one end, so you can stack them up, still pull out the ones you need, and keep your precious heels in mint condition.

"Wedges or stilettos?"

Wedges are more comfortable (think relaxed summer espadrille version) but stilettos are sexier (think high heels that give you long, long legs). Get a few of both.

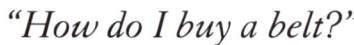

"How do I buy a belt?"

You don't need to buy one, you need (at least) three. Firstly, a wide belt made from battered leather: wear it slung low around your hips for a beachy/boho look. Secondly, a skinny belt to go into pant loops to smarten an outfit for the office or a party. Thirdly, a chunky belt in leather or patent: wear over a skirt or rain coat to pull in your waist and create serious curves.

"Which accessories work on bigger-busted women?"

Draw attention to your assets with a locket or long, chunky necklace.

"How can I accessorize? I've got big hips."

The key for pear shapes is to draw attention away from the hips. Wear shoulder bags with short straps that hang just below the armpit rather than at hip height. Jewelry should be worn on your upper half and low-slung belts should be avoided.

"Should your purse match your shoes?"

That approach is all very oldschool. The new rules say that clashing is the new matching, so team your red patent Mary Janes with an oversized, purple moc-croc clutch and pay homage to the art of the mismatch.

"How do I find sunglasses to suit me?"

As a general rule, you need to balance your face by choosing glasses of an opposing shape. So, round faces look good in angular glasses, square faces suit rounded ones, and oval faces can get away with pretty much anything.

"How do you buy pearls?"

Peals never come in perfect rounds, but the more circular they are, the more desirable they become. Look for pearls with a shiny luster and a good concentration of color near the drill holes.

"Is there a way I can make my face look slimmer?"

Go for longer earrings to elongate your face. Circular or hoop earrings should be saved for long, thin head shapes.

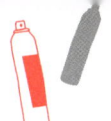

"How can I hide my greasy hair?"

Hairbands have been all over the catwalks during the last few years and provide an excellent coverup. If you have a large, deep head, go for broad bands, but stick to skinny or thinly braided ones if your crown is smaller.

"What's the best way to grow out bangs?"

Braid a few pieces of elastic together or use a skinny hairband to pull it off your eyes and use hairpins the same color as your hair to pin stray bits back.

"How can I create new looks from the clothes I already have?"

Instead of building an outfit then looking to accessorize, do it the other way around. Choose your best piece of jewelry, purse, or pair of shoes, and pick out a color, pattern, or shape that will work in your clothes.

"Can short people wear hats?"

Hats are an oft-neglected accessory that can turn an outfit around. Shorter people should avoid hats with wide brims (they'll look like a mushroom) and go for hairpieces and decorations or mini toppers that perch jauntily on the side of your head and add height to your overall stature.

"How do I know what body shape I am?"

As a general guide, apples have broad shoulders, carry weight on the bust and stomach and have slim legs. Pears have a small chest, thin arms, narrow shoulders, curvier hips and gain weight easily on the bum. String beans are straight up and down with a small bust and hips, and hourglasses are curvy with a full bust and hips but a narrow waist.

"How do I dress up an hourglass figure?"

Make like a 1950s housewife and go for full, knee-length skirts with a flair, nipped in by a belt to show off your slim waist and top with a sweetheart neckline. Some Mary Jane heels will complete the look.

"How can I dress to make my legs look longer?"

Dressing is all about proportion. You can go the traditional route of wearing some skyscraper-high heels under high-waisted, wide-legged, or boot-cut pants that reach almost to the floor. Or go for dresses with an empire line (with a seam just below the bust), or a baby-doll silhouette (flare outward from the bust). By raising your waistline, your legs will automatically look longer.

"Are high heels the best way to make my legs look longer?"

There is nothing more silly than a short woman wearing heels as big as she is, so no. Every women has a *perfect heel height* (PHH) that complements the natural arch in their foot, improves their posture, and maximizes their height. How to find this is trial and error.

"What's the best way to slim my thighs?"

If you've got thunder thighs, go for wide-legged slacks that skim your widest part and balance out your skinnier calves. Skirts-wise, pick flared shapes that kick out from the waist and drop to the knee. Never ever go for bubble or tulip shapes, which will exaggerate your problem area.

"Is there a way I can make my calves look thinner?"

High heels are the fastest route to less chunky calves; go for pointy toes over round ones.

"How can I make myself look taller?"

In addition to your skyscraper heels, wear long accessories like a skinny scarf or a slimline clutch bag to elongate your silhouette.

"What kind of top will balance out my big hips?"

Choose wide and boat-neck tops, which will add width to your shoulders to counteract that of your hips.

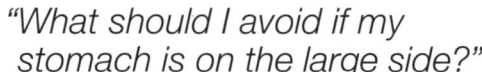

"What should I avoid if my stomach is on the large side?"

Never use a tight belt to try and hide the area: the effect will be the opposite. Draw attention upward with necklaces, earring, or brooches instead.

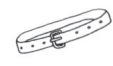

"How can I lose pounds off my waist in seconds?"

Short of holding your breath for the day, your best option is control pants, such as Spanx by Sara Blakely. These hold in the waist to give you back your curves and are often seam-free for a smooth finish under clothes.

"What's the key to dressing for large figures?"

Tight clothes may overexpose your bulges but don't be tempted to go for baggy clothes, which will make you look like you're wearing a tent. Go for something in the middle with clothes that skim, rather than cling to, the body.

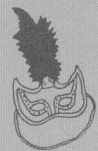

"How can I hide my big tummy?"

If you've managed more chocolate bars than sit-ups recently, pick empire-line tops that are tightest below the bust rather than over the belly. Fitted tops that flare over the hips will also act as a good mask. If you've got a good bustline, draw the attention down with a V-neck.

"What's the best way to dress a pear shape?"

If you're bottomheavy, the key is to create a strong shoulder line. Avoid flimsy spaghetti straps and go for a slash-neck, then avoid anything that clings to your bottom. Dresses and skirts that skim over and flare out at the hips should do the trick.

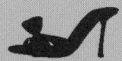

"How can I soften broad shoulders?"

Create a more feminine look with button-down shirts and blouses that show a bit of neck. Avoid sweetheart-line necks and shoulder pads, of course.

"How do I flatter my big shoulders and bust?"

Use V-necks to draw the eye down toward your navel, emphasize your waist with wrap-around tops or dresses (Diane Von Furstenberg is the queen of the wrap dress) and choose tailored skirts or slacks to bring attention to your legs. Avoid crew necks and double-breasted jackets at all costs.

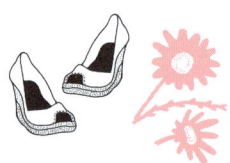

"How can busty types get a sleek silhouette?"

This is all about defying gravity. A good bra is key to stop your bust melting into your stomach. Thin fabrics also create lift (rather than chunky ones, which add bulk) and plain clothes aren't weighed down by busy patterns.

"Is there a way I can streamline my silhouette?"

Have a bra fitting: women's breasts change shape and size over time and a wellfitting bra will do wonders for your figure.

"How can I slim my flabby arms?"

If your arms are less shapely than you'd like, wear thin, delicate jewelry to draw attention to your wrists and away from your sagging upper arms.

"Which tops will hide my sagging underarms?"

Avoid anything with puff or elasticated sleeves and go for three-quarter or longer sleeves in light, floaty fabrics to draw attention to your daintier wrists.

"How can I hide a sagging neck?"

Go for turtlenecks, open-neck shirts with large collars, or tie a silk scarf to conceal the droop.

"What can I wear to make my neck look longer?"

Tops with cowl, scoop, or V-necks will draw the eye downward and create a streamlined effect.

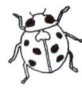

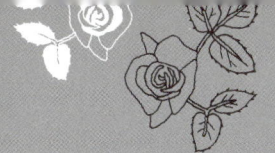

"What should I wear to hide a crêpey chest?"

Instead of baring your décolletage, go backless. It's just as sexy but not as saggy.

"What works on a petite frame?"

The key is to break up your body. Go for cropped jackets, three-quarter length sleeves (but never cropped pants), and tight jeans or fitted skirts. Look for detailing (buttons, zips, decorated hems, and so on) and you can afford to go big on accessories to add interest to your look.

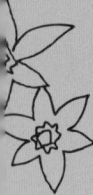

"How do you find a print that works on small frames?"

Every season brings a new wealth of prints, be they mini florals, macro flowers, ethnic, polka dots, or abstract. Despite traditional advice warning petite women against big prints, small frames can get away with them by wearing them on one item (a blouse always works well) rather than head-to-toe. Layer it with a one-color jacket or cardigan to stop it from swamping you.

"What's the best way to balance out my long body?"

If your legs are outshone by a longer torso, balance out your silhouette with high-waisted slacks worn to the ground over high heels. Shorter tops with horizontal strips will help, and a skinny belt worn over the top tucked into the slacks will elongate your legs and truncate your long body.

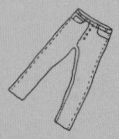

"How can I make my boyish figure look curvier?"

Do what designers do and play with proportions. Tulip and cocoon shapes will add volume to your bottom half, belts can accentuate your waist and a push-up bra will do wonders for your bust.

"Which colors will show off my tan?"

White will look cool, blacks sophisticated, pastels are good for day and hot pinks, turquoises, and yellows will look good at any time. For parties, gold will set off your bronzed limbs.

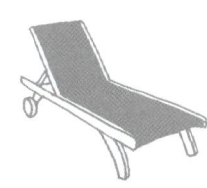
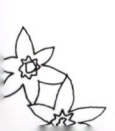

> *"I am about to get married for the second time. Now older, can I still go for the full flowing brides dress or should I pick something more classic and reserved?"*

Apart from resisting the urge to wear a blusher veil that covers the face, a style traditionally reserved for first-time brides, there is no reason why you shouldn't have fun selecting your dream dress for your second wedding. The options are endless, but take care to ensure the dress suits the tone of the ceremony.

"Matching accessories—still stylish or a fashion faux pas?"

Once upon a time it was considered a huge fashion crime should your hat, scarf, handbag, and shoes not match. These days, the matchy-matchy, homogenized look is often viewed as dated. Choose accessories that compliment rather than match each other.

> *"I need to find the perfect first date outfit that will leave a lasting impression and my date wanting more."*

There are a number of things to consider when choosing your first date outfit:

What you feel best in. Confidence is considered one of the most attractive traits, so wearing what you feel most desirable in will make you look and feel great, giving you a confident glow!

Your best features. It's important to choose items that enhance your best bits and disguise those you are least happy with.

Definitely don't:

Choose inappropriate shoes. As tempting as those killer heels may be, only wear shoes you can walk in—painful blisters and your date scraping you up from a heap on the pavement is definitely not a good look.

Flaunt too much flesh: Follow the age-old rule of not revealing both legs and cleavage to ensure your look stays sexy without crossing the line to trashy.

"Feminine, lace dresses are everywhere in the shops. How can I wear one without looking too girly?"

Add a touch of masculine tailoring. Team a pretty dress with a blazer in a darker, contrasting shade for a daytime look. In the evening, forgo the delicate and add a chunky pair of heels.

"I have a beautiful dress I wear during the daytime, but its gray. What can I do to stop it looking dull?"

Accessorize with playful jewelry in bold colors or go for a louder pair of shoes. In the colder months, wear a long sleeved t-shirt or pullover underneath in white, light blue, or baby pink to break up the dark tones.

> *"I have arrived at my work party and one of my colleagues has turned up in exactly the same dress as me. How do I prevent this happening in the future?"*

Unless you have a crystal ball it's unlikely you will be able to foresee this situation occuring beforehand, so try carrying a decorative scarf, a quirky pair of heels, or a stand-out necklace to slip on to make the look your own should history repeat itself.

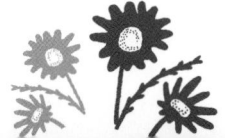

Travel tips

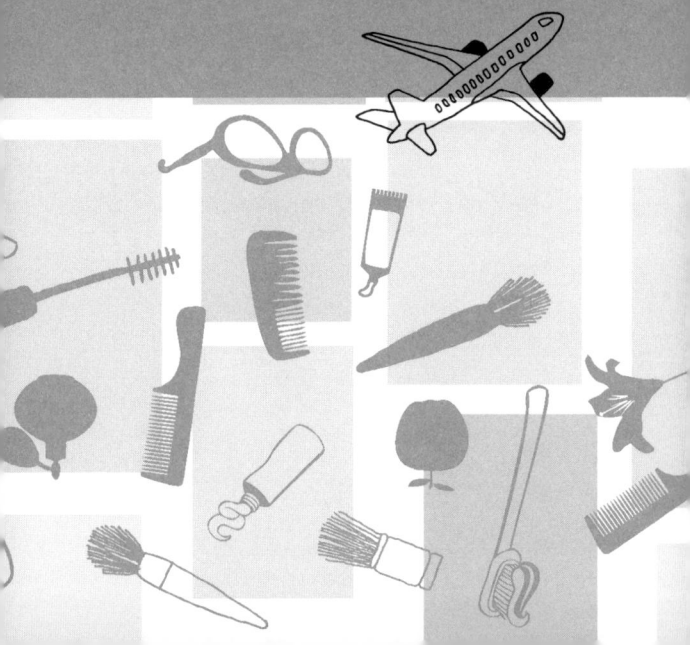

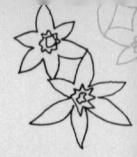

"How can I stop myself from feeling sick on the plane?"

Buy some ginger candies to suck. They will ease the pressure in your ears during takeoff and landing, plus quell your feelings of nausea.

"What are the essential beauty items I need for my hand luggage?"

- Make-up essentials (concealer, blush, mascara, lip balm)
- Toothpaste, toothbrush, and mouthwash
- Tissues and antibacterial wipes
- Cooling facial spray and moisturizer, to double up as hand cream
- Eye pads
- Water
- Saline nasal spray

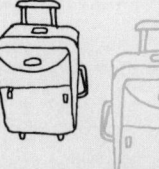

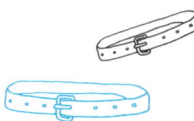

"What are the summer vacation luggage essentials?"

- Bikini or swimsuit
- Coverups such as kaftans or sarongs
- Linen or pure cotton slacks
- Sundress
- Evening dress
- Shorts
- Flip flops
- One pair of wedges or high-heeled sandals
- Sunhat
- Chunky/ethnic necklace or bangles
- One belt for slacks or a dress
- Long- and short-sleeve tops
- Knitted cardigan or sweater for cooler evenings

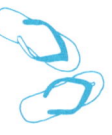
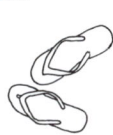

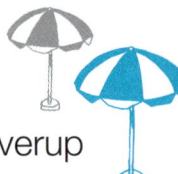

"What should I wear to coverup on the beach?"

If you're in your 20s, try a toweling dress or spaghetti-strap sundress; in your 30s, wear a sarong over a bikini or swimsuit for a chic look; for those in their 40s and above, go for a kaftan in a bright color.

"Where can I find stylish ski wear?"

Make like a celebrity and go for a designer label: Chanel do salopettes and even skis. But if it's a sporty look you're after, Quicksilver and O'Neill do a ski range.

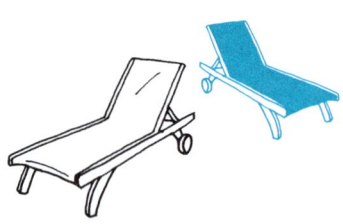

"What type of sunglasses are best for ski vacations?"

If you don't want to go for full-on goggles, pick wraparound shades. Not only will they stop sunlight and reflections from the snow from bouncing into your eyes at the side, they'll also give you more protection against crow's feet.

"What's the best make-up for poolside sunbathing?"

You want to look your best, but a full face of make-up will clog your pores and leave your foundation melting down your face. Wear a tinted waterproof moisturizer with SPF to kill three birds with one stone, then top with an SPF lip balm and some waterproof mascara.

"Should I change my make-up when I'm on vacation?"

Even after you've applied your sunscreen meticulously, you should develop a tan. Darker skin can take bolder color, so pack some eye shadows and lip glosses similar to the ones you usually use, but a shade or two brighter for evenings out.

"How can I streamline my antiaging skin regime on vacation?"

No room for moisturizers, serums, night creams, peels, and brighteners? Pack a regular moisturizer and a small pot of grapeseed oil: adding a few drops will give you the youth-boosting benefits you need while you're away.

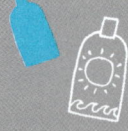

"What should a good vacation toiletries bag contain?"

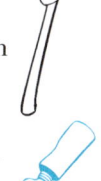

- SPF sunscreen, tinted foundation, lip balm and hairspray
- Aftersun or aloe vera for moisturizing
- Shampoo and conditioner (if not supplied where you are staying)
- Toothbrush and paste
- Tea tree oil for breakouts
- Citronella spray to ward off insects
- Nail polish, remover, file, and scissors
- Razor and a pair of tweezers for stray hairs

"How can I streamline my vacation toiletries bag?"

If your toiletries bag takes up half your luggage, simply leave it at home. Buy a range of products online from a site such as www.hqhair.com, and get them delivered to your hotel ready for when you arrive.

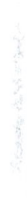

"What are the beauty essentials for a sailing vacation?"

Once you've got the wind in your hair, make-up will be the last thing on your mind. Ditch the mascara and go for products that offer protection against the elements, such as sun cream, SPF hair spray, hair detangler, and super-strong conditioner (you'll need it after all that wind and salty air), hand cream to ward off calluses if you're crewing, a gentle facial and body exfoliator to remove dry salt at the end of the day, plus after sun or aloe vera.

"How can I protect my hair in the sun?"

Hair burns just as skin does. When you're going in the sun, mix equal amounts of an oil-free SPF sun tan lotion with an oil-free hairspray, rub together in your palms and smooth over your hair.

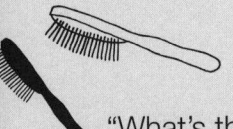

"What's the best way to protect my hair from chlorine?"

Because hair is porous, it will absorb the damaging chemicals in chlorinated water. To provide a barrier to this absorption, mix equal amounts of a leave-in conditioner and sun tan oil (make sure it is oil-based) in your palms, then slick over your hair for a by-the-pool wet look.

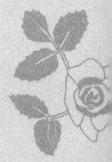

"How can I stop my hair from going brittle in the sun?"

Take a bottle of a super-conditioning mask with you and slather it onto your dry hair before going out in the sun.

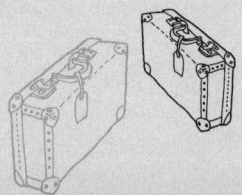

"What is a tan?"

The pigment melanin is produced by the cells in the skin and gives the skin its natural color. When exposed to sunlight, the skin produces more melanin to try to absorb the harmful UV rays, making it go darker.

"Does getting a base tan before I go on vacation protect my skin from sunburn while I am away?"

As tempting as it is to have a pre-vacation stint on the sunbed, don't. Although the sunlamp gives your skin the equivalent protection as an SPF 4, this is still far too low. Any change in the color of your skin is a sign of ultraviolet damage that can cause premature aging and skin cancer.

"Do I still need to wear sunscreen if I have dark skin?"

While it's true that dark skin provides some protection against skin damage, it is not a foolproof method of protection against skin cancer and premature aging, so yes.

"Is it true that sunscreens can actually harm your skin?"

Both PABA (padimate-O, also known as octyl dimethyl) and DEA (diethanolamine) are present in most sunscreens and have been linked to DNA damage and an increased risk of skin cancer. Other chemicals to avoid in your sunscreens are benzophenone, titanium dioxide, and parabens.

"What's the difference between sunscreen and sunblock?"

Sunscreens absorb UV rays chemically while sunblocks deflect them physically.

"What should I look for in a good sunscreen?"

SPF (sun protection factor) refers to the defense sunscreen gives against UVB rays, which cause sunburn. The SPF should be at least 15. A PA rating refers to the level of protection against UVA rays responsible for long-term skin damage. These will be marked as PA+ or PA ++: the more crosses, the greater the protection. Get a sunscreen with a broad spectrum that protects against both UVA and UVB, and contains avobenzone, oxybenzone, mexoryl, and zinc or titanium oxide.

"Do I need to wear the same amount of sunscreen when skiing as I would on a beach?"

High altitude rays pose as much damage to the skin as those at low altitude, so pick a high-factor sunscreen with protection against both UVA and UVB rays and pay particular attention to the nose, neck, and chin, which become especially vulnerable when the sun's rays deflect off the snow.

"What's the best sunscreen for older skin?"

With the wonders of modern technology, you can protect your skin from the sun and repair former damage. Sisley have developed the Sunleya Sun Protection, which contains both UVA and UVB protection, as well as antioxidants to ward off free radicals and damage to the skin cells' DNA.

"Do I need to wear sunscreen when it's cloudy?"

Eighty percent of UV rays can pass through cloud, so yes.

"Why do I tan more slowly than I used to?"

The production of pigment in your skin slows with age, so you take longer to build up that bronzed glow. Rather than fry yourself all day in the sun, stick to a fake tan to get the color you want.

"Are there any other ways I can protect myself from the sun, other than sun tan lotion?"

There are now pills based on antioxidants, which prevent the DNA damage caused to the skin by the sun's rays. However, these have not been developed sufficiently to replace sunscreen.

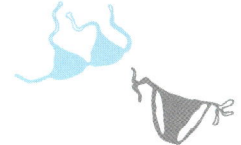

"Is there anything other than the SPF that I should look out for in a sunscreen?"

Choose a photostable product, meaning its filters do not break down in the sun.

"When should I apply sunscreen?"

About 20 to 30 minutes before you go out in the sun to allow the ingredients to bind to the skin.

"How does the sun visibly affect my skin?"

UV rays break down the skin's collagen and elastin, causing sagging. They also cause the skin to produce more melanin (pigment), which you see as dark age spots.

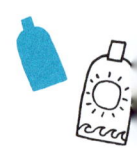

"Do I need to wear a sunscreen on my lips?"

With no melanin to protect them, lips are particularly vulnerable to sunburn. Wear a balm containing at least SPF 15 with UVA and UVB filters. Some lipsticks even contain a sunscreen nowadays.

"How can I make my skin less prone to sun damage?"

As well as using a good sunscreen with protection against UVA and UVB rays, leave out any products containing alcohol from your beauty regime. Alcohol makes the skin more photosensitive, leaving you vulnerable to sunburn.

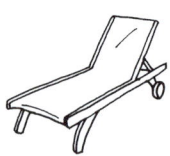 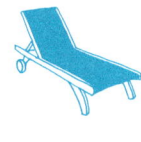

"How long before my vacation should I get a salon tan?"

Although they produce an even all-over tan, salon sprays can leave you looking a bit grubby. Have yours a couple of days before you leave: after a few showers the effect will be more natural.

"Are there other ways I can ensure my skin is protected on vacation?"

Take a PLE supplement. Made from a South American fern, *Polypodium leucotomos* tablets can help boost the skin's tolerance to the sun.

"Why do people with red hair burn more easily?"

Redheads produce a type of melanin called phaeomelanin, which provides poor protection against UV rays.

"Is getting a tan really that bad for my skin?"

Everyone may tell you that you have a healthy glow, but as well as the increased risk of skin cancer, tanning causes photo-aging, the main reason for wrinkles.

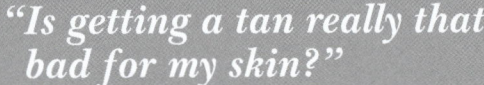

"How can I soothe sunburn?"

If you're not a fan of aftersun, apply some full-fat plain yogurt straight from the refrigerator onto the burnt area or add a cup of milk to a cool bath.

"Any other ideas for cooling sunburn?"

Splash a natural toner of cold green tea on it as often as you need to.

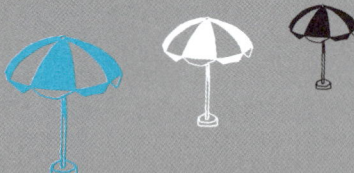

"How do I take the redness out of sunburn to stop it from ruining my evening party dress?"

To avoid looking like a lobster all night, seek out professional help. Most hotels now have a spa (or they'll recommend one nearby) where you can get a cooling body wrap to take the sting and redness out of your burns. Avoid wearing red that night and opt for cooling whites and icy blues to tone your skin down instead.

"How can I minimize the damage of sunburn?"

Add a few drops of peppermint oil to some aloe vera, cool it in the refrigerator and apply to the affected area.

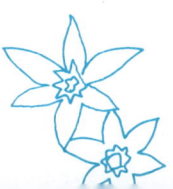

"How I can stop myself from getting eaten alive by mosquitoes?"

Reduce your intake of sugar (these pests love sweet blood) and start taking a B vitamin complex supplement (thought to act as a deterrent to mosquitos). Neem oil, when applied to the skin, is also thought to ward them off.

"How can I stop mosquito bites itching?"

Taking a vitamin C supplement and drinking nettle tea will both have the effect of a natural antihistamine. If you are somewhere hot with aloe plants, snap a leaf spine to release the sap and apply it to the sting to soothe the itch and reduce the swelling and redness.

"How can I cure my travel sickness?"

Carry a small bottle of peppermint or ginger oil in your handbag and inhale in slow, deep breaths when nausea strikes.

"What's the best way to prevent travel sickness?"

A Nevasic audio CD uses sounds, pulses, frequencies, and signals sent to and from the inner ear and the brain to lessen the feeling of nausea.

"How can I stick to my fitness regime on vacation?"

If there's no hotel gym, and you can't run outside, pack two essential fitness items: a skipping rope for a calorie-burning cardiovascular workout, and a Theraband (a wide rubber band) for resistance work to keep your muscles toned.

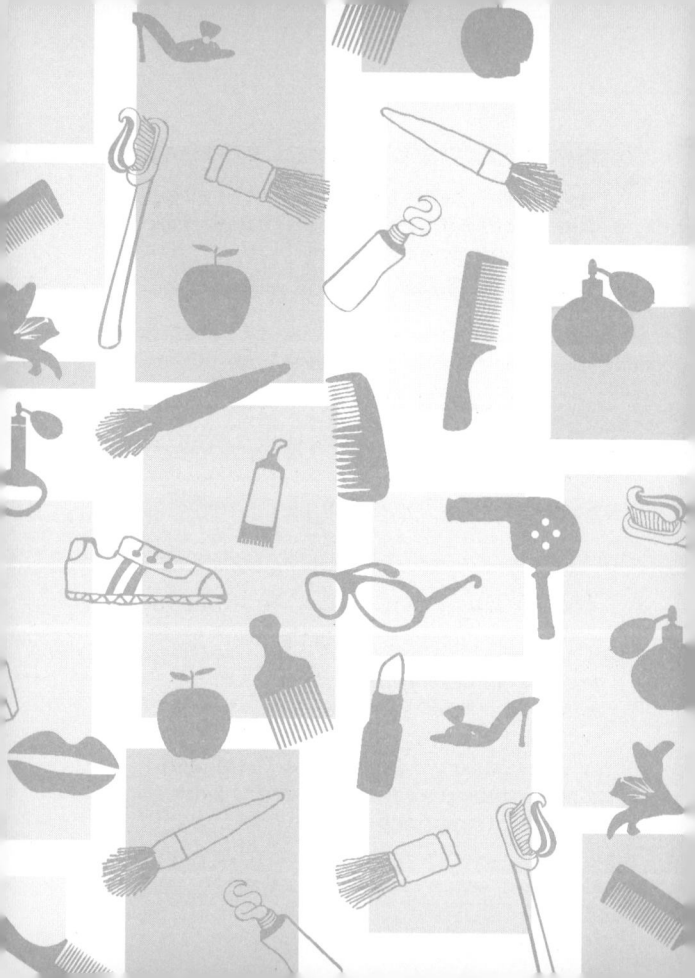

Myths & trivia

"What are the new weird and wonderful beauty trends?"

The Japanese have always been skin-care innovators. Now, women there are having the goldfish pedicure, where hundreds of tiny fish nibble at your feet to remove the dead skin. Keep a look out, too, for the bull serum hair mask and nightingale poo facial.

"Is there a natural way to remove earwax?"

Doctors advise patients against using cotton swabs in their ears because they can lead to perforations in the eardrum. Instead, warm some olive oil to body temperature and put a few drops in a waxy ear. Leave to settle for a minute, then tilt your head so the liquid oil can run out of the ear, bringing the wax with it. Rinse your ear gently with warm water.

"What's the difference between prebiotics and probiotics?"

Prebiotics nourish the good bacteria present in the gut, while probiotics provide it with the correct environment in which to thrive.

"Is eating raw food better for me?"

The Raw Food Diet is based on the belief that heating food above 240°F destroys the natural enzymes that help in the digestion and absorption of food. Basing your diet on uncooked, unprocessed fruit, vegetables, nuts, seeds, grains, and sprouts means you eat more nutrients without added harmful fats, salt, or sugar. Fans claim it will aid weight loss, clear your skin, boost your energy, and improve your digestion.

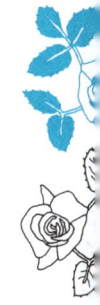

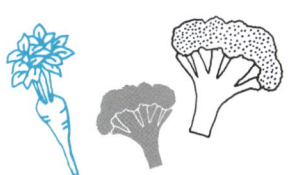

"Will eating too many carrots really turn my skin orange?"

Unfortunately, it's not an old wives' tale. The high concentration of beta carotene in carrots, squash, pumpkin, and other naturally orange foods can leave your skin with a yellow tinge, so vary your diet with fruit and vegetables of every color.

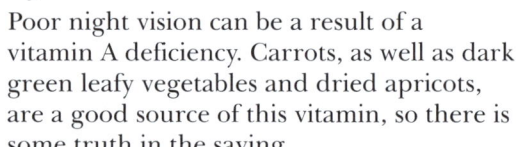

"Do carrots really help you see in the dark?"

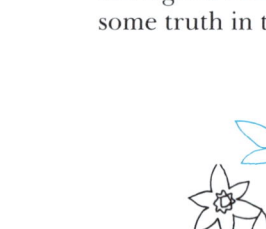

Poor night vision can be a result of a vitamin A deficiency. Carrots, as well as dark green leafy vegetables and dried apricots, are a good source of this vitamin, so there is some truth in the saying.

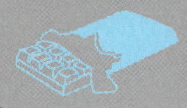

"Chocolate gives you acne: fact or fiction?"

Hormones and bacteria are the most likely causes of acne, not chocolate. However, the sugar content in many poor-quality chocolate bars can affect your skin adversely. Buy chocolate with 70 percent cocoa solids and a minimal amount of sugar instead. You'll minimize the risk of breakouts and give your body an added antioxidant boost.

"Is there really such a thing as beauty sleep?"

The need for getting your eight hours is no myth. Not only does sleep give the body a chance to recover from the day's activities, it's also a time for the cells to repair themselves. Getting a good night's sleep really can improve your skin's muscle tone and appearance and keep you looking younger for longer.

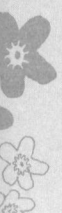

"What is Elizabeth Arden's real name?"
Florence Graham.

"When was deodorant invented?"
In 1888 by Mum.

"What do celebs use in the bath?"
Anyone whose skin is often on show doesn't risk using soap and chemical-based products that cause irritation and dryness. Instead, do as *Desperate Housewives* star Teri Hatcher does and add antioxidant-rich red wine to your bath.

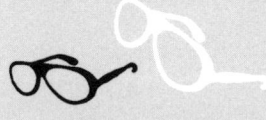

"Whose is the most requested celebrity body by cosmetic surgery patients?"

A survey by the Beverly Hills Institute of Aesthetic and Reconstructive Surgery showed that whether it's J Lo's bum, Angelina Jolie's pout, or Scarlet Johansson's bustline, the trend among plastic surgery patients is to pick and choose from stars' body parts rather than go for their look overall.

"What crazy procedures can cosmetic surgeons now carry out?"

A recent trend among plastic surgery fans is the umbilicoplasty, which reshapes the belly button to the patient's desired look.

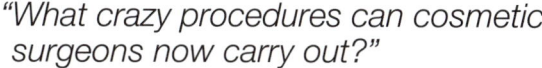

"Where does the term plastic surgery come from?"

From the Greek word *Plastikos*, meaning to mold or reshape.

"When did people first start having plastic surgery?"

Although it developed in leaps and bounds after World War II as a means of treating the wounded, the earliest incidences date back to ancient India over 3,000 years ago when physicians began using skin grafts for reconstructive work on the body.

"How much hair do we have on our bodies?"

We have hair everywhere except on the palms, soles, or your feet, nails, eyeballs, and lips: about five million hairs overall.

"Does shaving hair make it grow back thicker?"

To all those women who have long feared the razor blade, rest assured it's a myth. The color, thickness and distribution of body hair depends largely on genes and hormones. Your hair may look thicker as it grows out of the stubble phase, but it isn't.

"What's the difference between epilation and delipation?"

The former removes hair from the skin's surface (shaving, dissolving, and so on), while the latter removes it from beneath the surface (plucking, waxing).

"Why don't men get cellulite?"

The network of fibers that holds pockets of fat is different in a man's skin, plus men are less prone to storing fat overall due to their levels of testosterone.

"I started sunbathing young. Is it too late to start applying sunscreen?"

Although research claims that as much as 20 percent of sun damage is done before the age of 18, it's never too late to start protecting your skin with SPF and a vitamin C-based product to help rectify some of the damage.

"Why do I have dead skin?"

Every cell in the body is constantly dividing to form new ones. Of the many layers of skin, the cells in the lower part of the dermis are multiplying, pushing cells upward as more are made. The older, dead, cells are pushed to the surface. As we get older, our cells take longer to renew.

"How much skin do we lose?"

We shed between 30,000 and 40,000 skin cells every minute.

"Will applying oil make my skin greasy?"

If you want to keep your skin moisturized without looking like you've fallen into an oil slick, essential oils are the answer. Unlike vegetable oils, they contain no vegetable fat so are nongreasy.

"What's the best way to care for oily skin?"

Contrary to popular opinion, you should use an oil-based cleanser to dissolve excess sebum, then apply an oil-free moisturizer to leave you shine-free when made up.

"I have shiny skin around my nose, chin and forehead: does this mean I have oily skin?"

Shine in these areas, know as the T-zone, indicates normal skin. If you're getting shine on your cheeks only a few hours after applying make-up, that's the sign of an oily complexion.

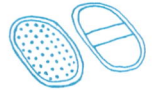

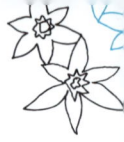

"Why do I get breakouts when I'm stressed?"

Stress stimulates our adrenal glands, leading to an increase in oil production. This in turn stops dead skin cells flaking off naturally, so pores become blocked and acne-producing bacteria multiply.

"Does the sun help dry out acne?"

While soaking up the rays may cause an initial improvement in your acne, in the long term it will only damage the skin cells and aggravate the condition.

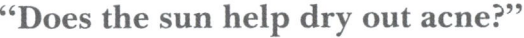

"Does toothpaste really help banish acne?"

An old wives' tale, I'm afraid. The menthol in toothpaste does have a drying effect, but it also contains fluoride and tartar-control agents, which can irritate the skin and make acne worse.

"What exactly are blackheads?"

These pesky problems are the result of oil in the pores oxidizing and turning black.

"Does my skin have any natural protection?"

The skin has a clever thing called the "acid mantle," an oily film sitting on the uppermost surface that helps kill bacteria and prevent damage from environmental impurities.

"What does pH stand for?"

Potential of hydrogen. It's a measure of the hydrogen ion concentration of a substance, what we know as acid or alkali. On the pH scale, 0 is extremely acidic, 7 is neutral and 14 is strongly alkaline.

"How may pores does the average woman have on her face?"

Twenty thousand.

"What's the natural pH of my skin?"

Most people's skin is between 4.5 and 5.5, so a little acidic.

"What are open pores?"

Pores are openings that let oil flow to the surface. When they become blocked by dead skin and other debris, they appear larger and therefore open.

"Was I just born with tricky, sensitive skin?"

You may well have been, but skin also changes throughout our lives with age, hormones, and other factors. So your skin may clear up and someone else who has had perfect skin all their life may experience problems later on.

"What's the best way to add moisture to my skin?"

Contrary to popular belief, moisturizers trap moisture in the skin, rather than adding more to it. Drinking plenty of water and eating fruit and vegetables can keep your skin healthy from the inside, leaving your moisturizer to work its magic on the outside.

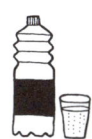

"Is it true that you should apply moisturizer to damp skin?"

New research suggests that instead of trapping extra moisture into the skin, applying hydrating creams to the skin when it's still damp can actually dilute the product and lessen its effectiveness.

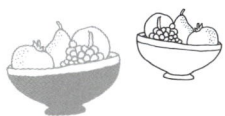

"Can I prevent wrinkles without cosmetics?"

Try taking a collagen supplement to help boost your complexion, improve the appearance of cellulite, and keep your hair and nails looking healthy too.

"Men get off lightly when it comes to aging. Or do they?"

A review has found that men may actually need higher doses of Botox to erase their wrinkles than women, due to their higher muscle mass. So it's not all bad being a woman.

"What do Hollywood starlets use on their faces?"

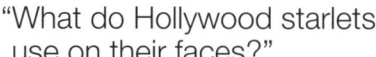

Anything can happen in Hollywood. Celebs have owned up to using skincare products containing placenta proteins. Makers of the products claim they are loaded with minerals, antioxidants, and amino acids to help replenish degenerating skin.

"Will facial exercises prevent me from getting wrinkles?"

Contrary to popular belief, some dermatologists claim that excessive use of the muscles around the eyes, forehead, and mouth can actually increase your chances of developing lines in these areas.

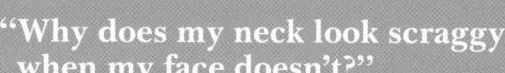

"Why does my neck look scraggy when my face doesn't?"

In our pursuit of eternal facial youth, we all too often neglect other areas. Unfortunately, our necks can give away our age. Not only is neck skin continually moving and stretching, but it has far fewer oil glands than the skin on our faces, leaving it prone to dryness and visible crêping.

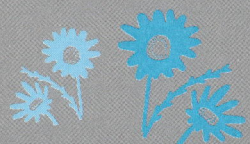

"My mother's skin has aged badly. Does that mean that mine will too?"

Genetics determine factors such as pore size, skin tone, and texture, but it's your lifestyle (whether you smoke, drink, remember to apply sunscreen, and eat a healthy diet) that will really determine the rate at which your skin ages.

"Does make-up provide any protection from environmental damage to the skin?"

When you trowel on your foundation and add a layer or two of blush and concealer, it may look like a mask, but it isn't. Make-up offers no shield to pollutants in the air or the sun's rays unless it has a SPF (sun protection factor) or EPF (environmental protection factor).

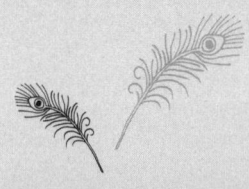

"When did women start using foundation?"

In Elizabethan times, a pale skin was a sign of nobility. The upper classes used a poisonous mixture of white lead and vinegar to make their faces completely white and cover the signs of aging.

"How extravagent can a beauty cream really get?"

For those who have got money to burn, La Prairie's Jewelled Skin Caviar Luxe Cream contains caviar proteins and comes in a bottle studded with Swarovski crystals.

"What was the first lipstick to come in the bullet-shape we still have today?"

Guerlain's Don't Forget Me.

"How much lipstick will I get through in a lifetime?"

The average woman uses 4 to 9 lb, and it's one of the items most frequently shoplifted.

"What traditionally gives lipstick its red color?"

The colorant carminic acid is extracted from boiled insects.

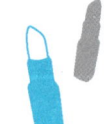

"When was the first indelible lipstick invented?"

Hazel Bishop of New Jersey began experiments in her mother's kitchen in the 1940s and brought the first smear-proof lipstick to market in 1950.

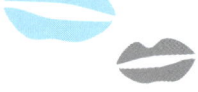

"Why do lips get chapped?"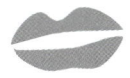

Lips lack the protective outer layer of skin (the epidermis) that covers the rest of our bodies, meaning the blood vessels are more visible and they appear pink. This lack of protection and the fact that they have no hair follicles or oil glands makes them particularly vulnerable to chapping.

"Is chewing gum good or bad for your teeth?"

The general consensus is that chewing gum, as long as it's sugar-free, can help prevent tooth decay. The increased amount of saliva produced as a result of chewing helps neutralize the acidity and clear the mouth of stray food particles. Xylitol, a sweetener in most gums, also reduces the number of Streptococcus mutans *bacteria in the mouth, which can cause tooth decay.*

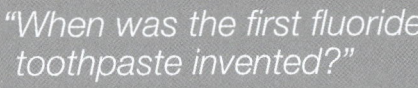

"When was the first fluoride toothpaste invented?"

In 1955 by Crest.

"What's a normal number of hairs to lose each day?"

The average person loses around 75 hairs a day as part of the natural cycle, but please don't start counting!

"I seem to lose a fair bit of hair every time I brush. How come I'm not bald?"

A hair grows for between three and five years before it reaches fulllength, goes into a resting phase and then falls out. Each follicle has a different growth and resting cycle so that different strands fall out at different times and you keep a full head of hair.

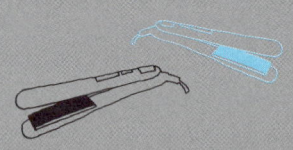

"Do we all have a similar number of individual hairs on our heads?"

The average person has 100,000 hairs. Blondes usually have the most (about 120,000), redheads the least (90,000) and brunettes come somewhere in the middle.

"Do I have the same strands of hair for life?"

No. It is likely your entire head of hair will be replaced ten times during your lifetime.

"Does all the hair on our heads grow at once?"

At any one time, 90 percent of your hair is growing and 10 percent is resting.

"Is chewing my hair dangerous?"

People who develop a habit of eating their hair are said to have a condition called "trichophagia." Because the acidic conditions of your stomach cannot break down the hair, it can form a ball and cause irritation or ulcers, which may eventually have to be removed by surgery.

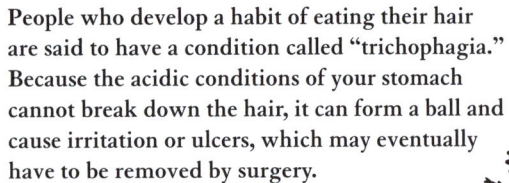

"Why do some people have straight hair and others curly?"

No matter how many times you straighten or perm your locks, your natural curl (or lack of) is determined by the shape of your hair shaft and the curve of the hair follicles in the skin. Examined under a microscope, straight hair looks round or oval and curly hair looks flatter. Straight hair generally has a straight follicle and curly hair a curved one.

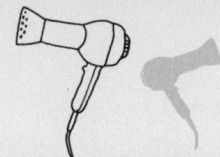

"Where did hairdryers come from?"

Alexandre Godefoy invented the first one in 1890, based on the concept of an early vacuum cleaner.

"Does cutting your hair make it grow faster?"

Sorry, but no. Regular hair appointments will help prevent splits and keep your hair looking healthier overall, but they won't make it grow faster.

"Is brushing your hair 100 times a day really good for it?"

You'll break your hair, pull it out, and irritate your scalp, so no.

"Why does our hair go gray?"

The cells at the base of the hair follicle stop producing the pigment that gives it its color.

"Is it true that washing my hair every day will make it dry?"

According to the old wives' tale, daily shampooing will somehow strip your hair of its natural oils. According to hair maestro Philip Kingsley, however, it is the hair's moisture level rather than oil flow that controls whether it's dry or not. In fact, the right shampoo can actually help to moisturize your hair.

"How can I repair split ends?"

Unfortunately, you can't. Cut them off, then try to prevent further ones by using moisture-rich conditioners and masks, and not straightening your hair to a cinder.

"What's the point of caring for my hair if it's dead?"

The fact that hair is physiologically dead means we can cut it without it hurting or bleeding. It is made from a protein called keratin and grows from follicles in our scalps. Each follicle has its own nerve, muscle, and supply of blood. Without proper nourishment from the blood capillaries, our hair suffers. Frequent shampooing stops a buildup of dirt on the scalp, and conditioner detangles, smoothes the hair, and adds shine.

"Can I make my hair thicker?"

We are all born with a specific number of hair follicles, which stays the same throughout our lives. The thickness of our hair depends on the size of the follicle, so while products can make it look fuller and more volumized, it won't actually be any thicker.

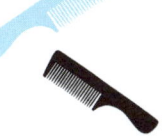

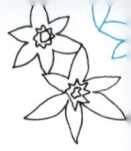

"Is greasy hair really the cause of dandruff?"

Dandruff is unrelated to oiliness and is actually caused by having a very dry scalp, a skin condition called psoriasis, or a yeastlike fungus.

"Does hair get used to the same shampoo?"

The widely touted belief that hair becomes resistant to the same shampoo over time is a marvel of modern marketing. An improvement in your hair after changing products is more likely to mean that your hair has changed, or that you were using the wrong product for your hair type in the first place.

"How does shampoo differ from conditioner?"

While shampoo opens up the hair cuticle in order to cleanse it, conditioner closes it down afterward.

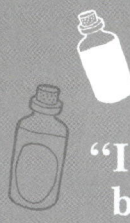

"Is baby shampoo really better for my hair?"

This shampoo is designed not to sting. It has no superior cleaning or conditioning properties.

"When was hair dye invented?"

Eugene Schueller, the French chemist who founded L'Oreal, created the first synthetic dye in 1907.

"Why is gray so much harder to dye than other hair colors?"

Colorists often call it *resistant gray* due to its coarse texture, which allows it to withstand dye.

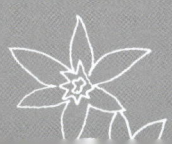

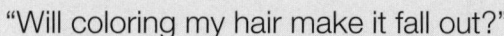

"Will coloring my hair make it fall out?"

Dyeing your hair (especially with bleach) may make it more prone to dryness and breakages, but there is no scientific evidence to suggest that it results in hair loss. In fact, bleach can sometimes make the roots seem plumper, making your hair look thicker overall.

"Where does the natural hair in hair extensions come from?"

People with very long hair (often in developing countries) can sell their hair to be used as extensions. So, no, it doesn't come from dead bodies!

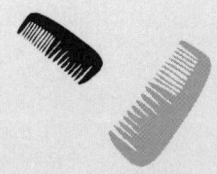

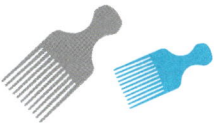

"Where did the perm come from?"

You might think that the perm was an 80s invention, along with power suits and shoulder pads. However, the first perm machine was developed in the early 1900s using electricity and various liquids to create curl in the hair.

"Will wearing nail polish damage my nails?"

Nail polish can actually stop your nails from breaking. Just don't pick when your polish chips or you'll remove nail cells.

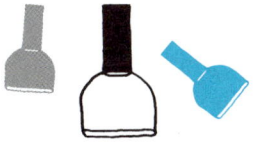

"Why are nail tips white?"

Nails appear pink due to the blood running through the capillaries in the skin beneath them. The tip overhangs the skin and has no pigmentation of its own so appears white.

"Does nail polish remover damage your nails?"

In short, yes. Touchup chips with more polish rather than using remover over the whole nail. When you want to change your polish, use a remover that is free from acetone, which dries the nails.

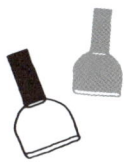

"When was nail polish first used?"

It can be traced back as early as 3000 B.C.E. in China, a mixture of beeswax, egg whites, and gelatin. The Ancient Egyptians used henna to dye their fingernails.

"What affects the rate of growth of my fingernails?"

As strange as it sounds, the longer the finger, the faster the nail grows!

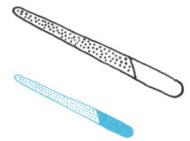

INDEX

A
accessories 344–7, 382, 384
aches and pains:
  treatment for 187
acne 215, 252–3, 310, 311, 312, 319
  on back 75
  blackheads 76, 77, 316, 421
  chocolate and 413
  concealing 13, 77
  facemasks for 76
  on hairline 105
  preventing 14, 76, 104
  reducing 14
  and stress 420
  in sun 420
  squeezing 104
  treatments 77, 214, 256
  under make-up 14
  using toothpaste on 420
  zapping: gadgets for 105
age spots 53
AHAs *see* alpha hydroxy acids
alcohol: types 43
Alexander Technique 300
allergies: to Botox 230
alpha hydroxy acids (AHAs) 50–1, 64, 99
amino acids 56
animals: products tested on 47
ankles: depuffing 246
anthotherapy 174
antiageing products 49–50, 50, 55–6, 70, 103, 218
antioxidants 49, 54, 67, 71, 283
anxiety: overcoming 290
apitherapy 169

Arden, Elizabeth 414
arms 297, 377
aromatherapy massage 182
arthritis treatments 176
Ayurveda 179–80

B
back 75, 77, 298
baineotherapy 177
bath salts: making 248
baths 248–9, 256, 289, 414
beach: covering up on 390
beauty creams: luxury 427
beauty products:
  indispensable 46
beauty sleep 413
beauty treatments: new 410
belts 366
bikinis 356–7, 358
black-tie events 342
blackheads 76, 77, 316, 421
blepharoplasty 215
blisters 267
bloating 275, 284
blowdrying 33, 89, 117, 120, 121, 122, 123–4
blueberries 308
blush 17, 141–3
body brushing 100
body odor 244, 289
body shape 370
body wrap 171
boobs *see* breasts
boots 364, 365
Botox 52, 222, 224–7, 228–30
boyish figure 381
brachioplasty 236
bras 349, 360
breakouts *see* acne

breasts 174, 299
  augmentation 238–40, 241
breath: bad 205
breath fresheners 23
brightening agents 69
bronzer: applying 135
brossage 187
bruising: preventing 297
brushes:
  hair 89–90
  make-up 21, 45, 96
bubble bath: making 249
burns 266, 267
bust: clothes 343, 350, 376
bust wrap 174
busty figure: clothes 377
butt facial 167
butt lift 237

C
caffeine 80
calcium 319
capillaries: broken 214
carbohydrates 278
carbon-neutral treatments 177
cardio workout 296
carrots 412
cashmere: care 346
cellulite 58, 102, 165–7, 306, 417
ceramides 60
cheeks:
  bones: accentuating 143
  broken capillaries on 214
  flushed: disguising 144
chemical peels: alternatives 213
chest:
  acne on 77

crêpey: hiding 379
  keeping firm 55
chewing gum 429
chicken skin 78, 297
chili peppers 70
chocolate 177, 273, 413
cleansers 69, 72–3, 97
cleavage:
  keeping firm 55
  revealing 383
clothes:
  black: alternatives 345
  for busty types 377
  celebrity styles 338
  colors 341, 342–3, 345, 352
  creating new looks 369
  designer: at bargain prices 339
  finding style 340
  for long-legged look 371
  for slimmer look 373–5
  storing 346
  to make bust bigger 343, 350
  vintage 336
  wrap dresses 348
co-enzyme Q10 50, 54
coats: winter 356
colds 187
collagen 52, 56, 67, 219, 424
colonic irrigation 287
complexion: flawless 133
concealers 127, 134, 138, 139, 146–7
conditioners 91, 127, 436
contour threading 212
copper peptides 67
cosmeceuticals 54
cosmetic surgery 208–10, 415
cosmetics 37–9

discontinued: finding 161
craniosacral therapy 181
cravings 168, 169, 281
cryogenic facial 191
crystal massage 185
cupping 188
cuticles: splitting 29

Dandruff 322, 436
day creams 66
deodorants 25, 244, 414
depilation 417
dermal fillers 217–23, 228
dermatitis 302
detoxing 285–7
diets 269, 281
dresses 100, 348–50
  gray 384
  lace 384
drinks 275, 306

Earrings 368
ears: stickyout 202
earwax: removing 410
eczema 302, 305
elbows 10, 101
elderberries 70
electrolysis 196
emollients 74
energy 240, 274, 278, 290, 293
environment 177
epilation 417
essential oils: safety 47
exercise 294, 296
exfoliating agents 10, 12, 50–1, 62, 64, 98, 99, 251, 254
exfoliation: before shaving 107
eye cream: natural 79

eye shadow 19, 21, 150, 151
eyebrow pencils 154
eyebrows 22, 109–11, 111, 165, 216, 314, 317
eyelashes 18, 20, 80, 152, 164, 195
eyelids: saggy 21
eyeliner 144, 149, 150
eyes:
  applying concealer 146–7
  bags under 146, 215
  bloodshot 317
  blue: accentuating color 144
  circles under 79
  gritty feeling 109
  healthy 316
  instant lift for 108
  lines under 256
  looking bigger 145
  looking farther apart 145
  looking wider 146
  make-up: lasting longer 151
  puffy 80, 257, 258
  radiant: achieving 258
  red: soothing 257
  rejuvenating 195
  shadows under 80, 147, 317
  smoky: achieving 153
  tired: refreshing 18
  under-eye area: perking up 259

Face:
  broken capillaries 312
  choosing products for 66–7
  cleansing 97, 253

INDEX

contoured effect 140
dark areas on 140
depuffing 99
dry skin on 12, 250
exercises for 425
hair on 99
massaging 98, 99
natural lift to 12
pores on 421
shading 144
slimming effect for 368
T-zone 419
toning 106, 195
using soap on 58
face peels 193
face-lifts 71, 196, 212–13, 224, 319
facemasks 68, 76, 252, 255
facial washes: for blackheads 77
facials 189–92
Fami (Fat Auto-graft Muscle Injection) 234
fangotherapy 181
fat (body) 277, 279
fats: good 275
feet 78, 237, 244–5, 286, 298–9
fingernails: growth 441
first date 383
fitness: vacation regime 407
flotation tanks 180
flu: recovering from 294
food: raw 411
forehead: lines on 194
formaldehyde 84
foundation 96, 99, 133–4, 135, 136, 139–41
earliest use 427
fragrances: in cosmetics 37
free radicals 55
fruit: benefits of 273
fungal infections 298

G
adgets 105–6
glow: healthy 135, 137
grazing: discouraging 279
gym 131, 334

H
air:
adding volume 92
after swimming 264
bed-head 119
blonde:
  changing to 87
  colored: reviving 265
  greasy roots 31
on body 416
breaking 327
brittle, colored 202
brown: adding shine 265
brushing 118, 433
bubble hair 321
buildup on 117, 263
care 435
chewing 432
chlorine protection 395
color stripping 201
combination: products for 92
conditioning 116, 263
curly: taming 118
cutting 433
daily loss 430
damage from styling tools 120
drab: refreshing 265
dry 320, 321, 324
dull 115, 262–3
dyeing: damage done 438
extensions 126, 203–4, 438
facial 99, 316
fine 123, 203
flyaway 31, 119, 122, 124
frizzy 31, 328
glossy look for 119
gray 327, 434, 437
greasy 31, 369
growth 431
highlights 125
improving 307–8
lank 30
long: smooth finish on 122
loss 322, 329
natural products for 88
number on head 431
oily 264
pampering 201
protecting from pollution 91
red: bringing out color 264
refreshing 32
removal: permanent 196–9
replacing 431
salon-colored: refreshing color 88
shampooing: daily 434
shaving: effects 417
smooth: blowdrying for 121
snacks good for 283
split ends 434
straight and curly 432
straightening 200
sun protection 394, 395
supplements for 323
taming 31, 118, 119
thickening 324, 435
thinning: preventing 326
treatments before big event 203
unruly 91, 122

washing 115, 116
see also hair styles
hair care products 88, 90, 202
hair dyes 92, 93, 437
hair masks: using 117
hair straighteners 89
hair styles/styling:
 air styling 200
 bangs 32, 120, 328, 369
 beachy waves in 120
 before big event 203
 blow-drying 33, 89, 117, 123
 changing 325, 329
 crimped look 124
 for fine hair 203
 highlights 125, 326
 for older face 325
 over stickyout ears 202
 to suit face shape 201
 tools 120, 121
 for younger look 328
hairbrushes 89–90
haircuts: bad 125
hairdryers 433
hands:
 aging 103
 dry 246, 302
 ink stains on 11
 keeping warm 299
 preventing irritation 247
 protecting from sun 103
 rejuvenating 236
 smooth: achieving 247
 softening 53
hangovers: avoiding 289
hats 370
hay fever 267
headaches: easing 287
heels: cracked 78
height: adding 300, 373

hemp oil 48
highlighter: applying 137
hips: clothes balancing 373
hourglass figure: dressing 371
human growth hormone 218
humectants 40
hypnopuncture 168

Indonesia: treatments 170
ingredients: safety 41–2
ink stains: on hands 11
insect bites and stings 268
iron: absorbing 278

Jackets: styles 354–5
jeans 352–4
jewelry 308

Kaolin 68
knees 10, 101
knitwear 343, 346
kohl 150

Lanolin 42
laser treatments 197, 213, 215, 234
legs:
 calf implants 237
 looking longer: clothes for 371
light therapy 214, 217
light-headedness 289
lip balm 23, 81–2
lip gloss 97, 155, 159
lipomassage 166
liposuction 233–4
lipozomes 60

lips:
 adding sheen 160
 chapped 429
 cracked 259
 filler alternatives 222
 hydrating 259
 looking fuller 23, 157, 158, 159, 220
 looking smaller 158
 moisturizing 260
 nude look 156, 158
 protection from sun 402
lipstick:
 applying 156, 159
 broken 22
 changing shade worn 160
 chemicals in 81
 choosing gloss or 155
 color in 428
 discontinued: finding 161
 for hair coloring 157
 indelible 428
 lasting longer 155
 lifetime's use 428
 for nude look 156
 red: softening effect 160
 shape 427
 testing color 156
 using liner 155
long body: balancing 380
lulur 170
lymphatic drainage massage 182

Magnesium 319
make-up:
 applying 129
 of benefit to skin 72
 brushes 45, 96
 day to night 48, 128
 essential item 15

experimenting with 132
eye 144–54
removing 258
for flawless complexion 133
fresh-faced look 136
getting out of rut 131
glitter 132
in gym 131
melted 46
minimum 129, 131
multitasking products 129
for natural look 138
oily patches on 17
for oily skin 138
patchy 255
permanent 210–11
protection provided by 426
for redheads 130
removing 59
reviving 16
for vacations 392
Mandara treatment 184
mascara 79, 144, 147–9
massages 98, 99, 182–6
melanin 53
men: aging 424
MesoGlow 221
metabolism 259, 291–2
microdermabrasion 192–3
micropigmentation 210–11
migraines 181
milia 192
minerals 277
miniskirts 351
moisturizers 60, 98, 252, 419, 423
mood: boosting 27, 294
morning boost 288
mosquitoes 406

mouth:
canker sores 266
cracks and sores 318
mouthwash: making 260
muscles: stiff 298
myotonology 195

Nail polish 27, 30, 84–5, 111, 112, 113, 439, 441
nail polish remover 440
nails:
brittle 261
cleaning 113
color 440
creating longer look 113
extensions: damage caused 164
filing 112
fungal infection 262
keeping dirt-free 28
keeping fake tan off 29
nourishing 61, 91
painting: time for 28
ridges on 330
shaping 112
snagged 28
stimulating growth 331
strengthening 331
white spots on 330
neck 378, 425
necklines: turtlenecks 344
nickel: reactions to 308
night creams 66
nose:
blocked 25, 288
looking smaller 300
raw: concealing 25

Older women: clothes 341
omega fatty acids 275, 303
onions: benefits of 281
organic products 39–40
overweight 278
oxygen facial 191

Pain relief 186
palm oil 38
Panthermal treatment 188
panties: showing 362
panty hose 361
parabens 41
paraffin baths 187
pear shape: dressing 375
pearls 368
pedicures 410
pentapeptides 56
perfumes 85–7, 108, 345
perms 439
petite frame: dressing 379–80
pH 421, 422
phytotherapy 170
pigmentation: uneven 69
Pilates 282, 291
pizzicchilli 183
plaque: minimizing 261
plastic surgery 415–16
pollution 61, 91
pores 96, 105, 315, 421
prebiotics 411
pregnancy 63–4, 175, 183, 225, 339–40
preservatives 43
probiotics 411
products 34–93
psoriasis 309
purse essentials 33
purse: matching 367

INDEX 447

Rashes: soothing 315
Rasul baths 179
raw food: eating 411
redheads 130, 403
reflexology 186
reiki massage 189
relaxation 180, 248
rolfing 185
rosacea 144
running: footwear 295

Sailing: beauty essentials 394
sales: shopping in 337
salon treatments: at home 106
saunas 178
scars: diminishing 266
scent *see* perfumes
scrubs: making 250
selenium 307
self-criticism: avoiding 300
sericin 309
serotonin 272, 278
serum 60, 91
shampoos 90, 91, 92, 93, 116, 436–7
shaving 107, 299, 417
shaving cream: substitutes 26
Shiatsu massage 184
shoes 336, 363–6, 372
shoulders 376
silhouette: streamlining 377
ski wear 390
skiing 391, 399
skin:
    absorbing antiaging products 56
    adding moisture to 423
    after flying 386
    aging 426
    Asian coloring 140
    benefits of chocolate to 177
    bleaching 10
    on body: dry 171
    boosting 307, 309
    brightening 10, 249
    care 71, 74
    changes in 422
    choosing cleanser for 72
    choosing products for 66
    dark: foundation for 141
    dead 418
    dry 59, 176, 250, 252, 310
    effects of sun on 401
    flaky: improving 303
    genetics and 426
    giving glow to 12
    hard, dry: food for 304
    healing 305
    healthy: nutrients for 304
    improving 70
    instant protection for 11
    irritated 59, 250
    large pores: foundation for 06
    make-up of benefit to 72
    mature 57, 253
    natural protection 421
    nutrients for 254
    oily 68, 138, 254–5, 311, 315, 419
    pick-me-up 15
    pre-bedtime checklist 100
    protecting 308
    from pollutants 61
    from sun 67, 402
    see also sunscreens
    puffy 310
    radiant 314
    scaly 187
    sensitive 62, 75
        removing hair from 198
    shedding cells 418
    shiny: cleanser for 69
    silky-smooth 102
    smooth 309
    snacks to boost 282–3
    tolerance to sun 403
    unblocking pores 105
    using stem cells for 57
    vacation care 392
    vacation preparations 386
    winter protection 65
    see also exfoliating agents; pigmentation
skin-lightening products 61
skirts 351
slacks 352
sleep 180, 248, 272, 413
smile 24, 233
snacks 282–3
soap 21, 58, 65
spas 172, 173–4, 175–6
spider veins 62
stains: on clothes 25, 26
steam rooms 178
stem cells 57
stomach:
    flat: achieving 301
    large: clothes to disguise 373, 375
    upset 274
stress 26, 284, 420
stretch marks 63, 301
styling wax 91
sugars: value of 274
sun 67, 396, 401, 420
sunbathing: make-up 391

sunbeds 396
sunburn 404–5
sunglasses 368, 391
sunscreens 397–401, 402, 418
superfoods 70
surfactants 40
sustainable sources: products from 48
sweatpatches 344
Swedish massage 182
swimsuits 357–9

Tan/tanning 396, 400, 404
  colors to show off 381
  fake 11, 29, 101–2
  salon: before vacation 403
  spray: time for 165
tattoos 128, 241
teeth:
  bleaching kits 83
  brightening 24
  chewing gum and 429
  decay: preventing 83
  face-lift 319
  flossing 114
  fruits kind to 320
  healthy: diet for 319
  sensitive 82, 318
  veneers for 233
  whitening 24, 231–2, 261
tester samples 45
Thai massage 182
thermage 194
thongs 362
thread veins 235
throat: sore 290
tiredness 284
tocopherol 74

toenails 30, 78
toiletries bag: vacation 393
toner: using 97
toning up 282, 291
toothache: soothing 320
toothpastes 83, 260, 420, 430
tops 373, 377
Traeger massage 185
travel sickness 407
treatments: using natural products 169
tropicarium 178
trytophan 272, 273, 278
tummy: toning 295
tummy tucks 235

Umbilicoplasty 415
underarms: sagging 236
underwear: eco-friendly 362

Vacations 386–94, 388–9
vaginoplasty 210
vegetables: benefits of 273
vegetarians 303
vitamins 50, 74, 79, 80, 277, 297, 308, 318, 320, 412
multivitamins 272

Waist: slim look 374
wardrobe:
  adding interest 334
  on budget 338
  mainstays 335
  reviving 339
water 276, 306, 307

waxing 197, 197–8, 199
weddings: dressing for 347, 382
weight: assessing 278
weight loss 168, 234, 279–81
white-tie events 342
winter glow 135
work party 385
wrinkles:
  eliminating 13, 51, 139, 194, 217–18, 231, 313
  exercises for 425
  foods advantageous to 276
  preventing 314, 424
  types 216

Youthful looks: keeping 293

Zinc 322, 330
zinc oxides 54
zips 345